Integrative Health Coaching

A Resource Guide for Navigating Complementary and Integrative Health

An Annual Publication of the Faculty and Graduate Students
Integrative Health Studies Master of Arts Program
California Institute of Integral Studies

Editor
Meg A. Jordan, PhD, RN, CWP, ACC, NBC-HWC
Department Chair and Professor

Foreword
John W. Travis, MD, MPH

2018 Edition

Published by Global Medicine Hunter,® 16 Club View Dr, Novato, California 94949
Jordan, Meg A.
Integrative Health Coaching: A Resource Guide for Navigating Complementary and
Integrative Health
ISBN- 978-0-9625882-5-9
ISBN-10: 0-9625882-5-3

    1. Health coaching. 2. Wellness coaching. 3. Integrative health coaching. 4. Coaching psychology. 5. Wellness. 6. Health promotion. 7. Integrative health. 8. Complementary medicine. 9. Integrative medicine. 10. Alternative medicine 11. CAM

Includes bibliographic references.

Printed in the United States of America.

Contents of this guide are taught in the master's degree program in the department of Integrative Health Studies and Integrative Health Coaching at the California Institute of Integral Studies, 1453 Mission St., San Francisco, CA. CIIS.edu (415) 599-6199.

Information in this manual is not intended to replace medical advice from a healthcare professional.

By participating in and/or using this course material offered by the California Institute of Integral Studies and Global Medicine Enterprises, Inc., you are acknowledging and agreeing that you are solely responsible for all aspects of the conduct of your business and your practice as a health advocate or coach, and that you are not sponsored or endorsed or otherwise affiliated with Global Medicine Enterprises, Inc. or the California Institute of Integral Studies. Neither Global Medicine Enterprises nor the California Institute of Integral Studies are responsible or liable in any manner whatsoever for claims or liabilities arising from the conduct of your coaching or health advocacy business; and both disclaim any liability, loss, or damages that may result from the conduct of your business or practice, and/or your use of such courses and materials, and/or the information, advice, and techniques embodied in such courses and materials.

The laws that define the practice of medicine or other healthcare fields specify that the provision of delineated services is reserved for provision by those who are licensed to provide such services. These laws vary from state to state, and the delivery of service is dependent upon specific circumstances that require independent judgment and decision making.

TABLE OF CONTENTS

FOREWORD: THE CURRENCY OF WELLNESS IS CONNECTION
John W. Travis, MD, MPH

It took me almost 40 years of working in wellness to see that my work could be summarized in only these six words: *The currency of wellness is connection.*

Types of Connection

My Wellness Energy System, which I began developing in 1977, shows how we're all connected through twelve different primary forms of energy—those that we take in and those that we express after transforming them. Our wellness is a direct result of how smoothly and well we manage our energies. The twelve chapters of the *Wellness Workbook* describe each form of energy shown on the Wellness Wheel, and the self-assessed Wheel gives a graphic picture of results when taking the Wellness Inventory (see chapter below).

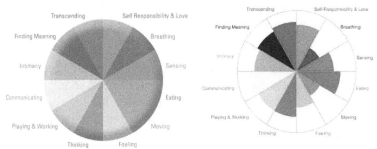

Wellness Energy Wheel   *Self-Assessed Wheel*

Modern Culture's Connection Bankruptcy

After I opened my Wellness Resource Center in 1975, I spent more than a decade working with people who were suffering from some of the many forms of disconnection that have become prevalent in our culture—depression, addiction, and chronic diseases of all sorts, including cancer and heart disease. The relationship between these ailments and their hosts' *lack of connectedness* in many areas of their life was not generally recognized—even by me at the time.

It was only in 1990, when a colleague pointed me to Jean Liedloff's *The Continuum Concept,* that I discovered this disconnection is not inherently part of the so-called "human condition," but rather is instilled in infants by modern cultural practices that unwittingly break the strong mother-infant bond.

Since this bond is the model that all subsequent relationships are built upon, it has lifelong consequences. Alienation is preventable! This led to my career shift to infant wellness, nearly three decades ago. I then realized its profound impact on adult wellness, and even upon the planet's wellness.

Since many of us aren't actively raising children, I struggled with how to incorporate infant wellness into my earlier work with clients and helping professionals. Whether or not we are actively raising children, many of us are unaware of the roots of childhood wellness, and how vital it is to meet children's early mammalian needs for connection.

This lack of connection during the primal period, or fourth trimester, later impacts our wellness as adults—ultimately contributing to the profound disconnection present in our culture. All of this disconnection can be traced back to our standard Western birthing and childrearing practices. It was only when I saw that their common denominator, or currency, is connection that the pieces of this puzzle joined up for me.

How Bad Is It?

Most of those who are raising children are too overwhelmed dealing with their own lives and immediate issues to consider yet another dimension of wellness. To understand both the underlying causes of disease and the value of wellness, we must first recognize the massive levels of disconnection around us—we are disconnected, on unprecedented levels, from ourselves, each other, our community/village, nature, and the sacred or divine (however perceived).

Yet few of us notice this near-bankruptcy, just as fish don't notice the water they are in. We're too close to it and have nothing with which to compare our experiences. Only by observing those few cultures that are still connected, can we begin to see how little of this currency we have in modern life.

In the US, and other "developed" countries, due to "modern" birthing/childrearing practices, we are now faced with four generations of adults who have been raised without their basic mammalian needs for physical and emotional connection being met—needs that have evolved, and been met, over millions of years.

As a result, most of us are now profoundly disconnected—yet largely unaware of it. I've been amazed when people who grew up in a connected culture, like Mexico, South America, Africa, or some Far Eastern countries, say that they can immediately see how disconnected our culture is.

Symptoms Indicating the Need for Full-Spectrum Wellness

Our culture is plagued with depression, addiction, violence, chronic illness, inauthenticity/"niceness," fear, rage, greed, fundamentalism, decaying social networks, war, and ecocide.

The cost of fixing these problems, *if a fix is even possible*, is probably beyond our means.

Prevention is the key. I believe Ben Franklin was on the right track, but his numbers were a bit off. I think an *ounce* of prevention is worth, not a *pound*, but more than a *ton* of cure. Yet billions of dollars continues to pour into treatment, while prevention is largely neglected.

Even more important than prevention is the active pursuit of wellness, which goes beyond the simple hope of preventing a negative condition. Wellness is much more thn avoiding an unwanted outcome—it offers a path to increase our zest for life.

Full-Spectrum Wellness

Full-spectrum wellness describes a multi-dimensional approach to addressing connection—the connections between our state of wellbeing and our:

- body, emotions, mind, and spirit,
- earliest life experiences and our health over our entire lifespan,
- family, friends, and community,
- personal and work lives, and
- environment—from our internal mind-chatter, to our home space, our neighborhood, our community, nation, culture, and the whole planet.

Increasing Wellness Levels

The first step to increasing the level of connection in our world is to work on ourselves. There are myriad excellent wellness programs to do this. Of course I'm biased toward the *Wellness Workbook*, and have continued my personal exploration of the ever-growing new approaches that have been appearing since its first edition in 1977.

These explorations have most recently led me to explore Jung's concept of the shadow and how we project it onto those around us whom we dislike or admire. Brené Brown's work on vulnerability and shame, largely in our shadow, helped me see how our level of personal connection is inversely proportional to our personal shame load, which is inevitably a part of growing up in a shame-based culture such as ours. Finding or creating supportive communities to replace the lost village or tribe is essential in healing our shame and increasing our wellness.

While most of the complementary and integrative health approaches described in this book fall under the treatment paradigm (see Illness-Wellness Continuum), the connection with the practitioner is essential for them to be effective.

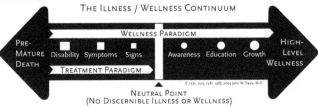

As a coach, your connection with your clients is paramount, so in their process of choosing any alternative/integrative practitioners, I hope you will instill the importance of their feeling a solid connection with the person when they make their choices.

Conclusion

Full-spectrum wellness is a multidimensional approach to enhancing connection—connection that extends from the individual to the collective, and ultimately the planet. Full-spectrum wellness enables us to explore and avoid many of the underlying connection-deficient causes of disease that manifest in individuals, families, communities, and the environment. Embracing and addressing the fundamental elements that characterize the connections inherent in full-spectrum wellness have the potential to raise the level of wellbeing on the planet.

This will create a world that honors connection and our one-ness. The ancients believed, and modern physics substantiates, *we are one.*

Resources

Alliance for Transforming the Lives of Children—aTLC.org.

Bowling Alone, Robert Putnam. Touchstone Books, 2001.

Connected Couples—Thriving Families—ConnectedAndThriving.org.

Connection Parenting, Pam Leo, Wyatt-MacKenzie. 2017.

The Continuum Concept, Jean Liedloff, Da Capo Press, 1986.

Daring Greatly: How the Courage to Be Vulnerable Transforms the Way We Live, Love, Parent, and Lead, Brené Brown, Avery, 2011.

Getting Real. Susan Campbell, HJ Kramer/New World Library, 2001.

Little Book on the Human Shadow. Robert Bly, Harper One, 1988.

Loving What Is. Byron Katie, Three Rivers Press, 2003.

Magical Child, Joseph Chilton Pearce, Plume, 1992.

Wellness Workbook. John Travis and Regina Ryan, Celestial Arts, 2004.

Wellness for Helping Professionals: Creating Compassionate Cultures. John Travis and Meryn Callander, Wellness Associates, 1990.

PREFACE

We are pleased to present *Integrative Health Coaching: A Resource Guide for Navigating Complementary and Integrative Health.* The guide is collaboratively written and published by the Advanced Health Coaching graduate students, faculty, and advisors in the Integrative Health Studies master's degree program at the California Institute of Integral Studies. Our master's program prepares students to enter the field of integrative health as coaches, practitioners, educators, researchers, administrators, and authors.

The integrative health and wellness coach employs advanced behavioral and integrative coaching strategies for helping clients move forward with their own desired goals, often in tandem with lifestyle medicine prescriptions from their healthcare providers. Individuals with chronic diseases are often challenged with getting the care they need to optimize their health and wellbeing. Working with a health coach can help them overcome those barriers, build confidence as they make healthier choices, and generally find a new "normal" as they cope with chronic illness through supportive approaches and resources in complementary and integrative health.

Whether coaches are asked to focus on adopting stress reducing techniques for managing pain or improving diet and exercise habits to better manage diabetes, they engage in a powerful client-centered process that helps individuals resolve ambivalence, identify key values and strengths, build resources and motivation, and move forward toward desired goals. The empowering journey is done at a pace that is attuned to the agenda, interests, capacity, energy, and preferences of the individual.

Most importantly, integrative health coaches go one step further by assisting clients as they explore the wide array of complementary, alternative, holistic, and integrative health tools; techniques; modalities; and whole healing systems available today—often a daunting task for someone struggling with compromised health and limited energy and finances. These holistic modalities and systems are often just what is needed to reduce stress, alleviate pain, and manage or improve overall health and wellbeing.

It is our intention that you find practical and valid information within these pages, and that this guide be a well-worn resource for communities, healthcare practices, companies, and coaches everywhere. We believe that wellness is a state of mind, as well as a day-to-day choice to live as mindfully and healthfully as possible, no matter what the physical capacity or diagnosis. The complementary and integrative health modalities and systems contained in this guide are in no way an exhaustive list of what is available, but they are among the most helpful and effective approaches that health coaches can share with individuals and their families. Our commitment is to keep expanding this guide as an online resource with more entries every year. We welcome your input.

To your health!

Meg Jordan, PhD, RN, NBC-HWC
Department Chair and Professor

ACKNOWLEDGMENTS

CIIS Integrative Health Studies Advisory Board
Michael Arloski, PhD
Hans Baer, PhD
Elliott Dacher, MD
Ricky Fishman, DC
Connie Grauds, RPh
Sally LaMont, ND, LAc
Richard McKinney, MD
Ricki Pollycove, MD, MA
Beverly Rubik, PhD
Len Saputo, MD
John W. Travis, MD, MPH
Katharine Weiser, MD, Shamanic practitioner

Contributing Editors
John W. Travis, MD, MPH
Rachel Lefkowitz, MA
Mary Beth Ferrari, MA
Molly Cumming

WHY COACHING FOR CHRONIC DISEASE?
Meg Jordan

You've probably heard of coaching, but not necessarily *integrative health coaching.* Coaches are experts in helping you change your perspective, behavior, hidden patterns, and beliefs that stand in the way of your goals or desired way of life. They help you accomplish the tough changes that you haven't been able to do on your own. What's more, they help you transform in a way that is personally meaningful and fulfilling. Whether that means you need to learn something new, or improve your performance, or adopt a new mindset—professional coaches have a plethora of tools to help you shed old patterns and unwanted habits, experience breakthroughs, and write a new chapter for your life.

Health and wellness coaches are specialists in the coaching field because they not only have to excel in the coaching process and powerful coaching dialog, but they need to be experts in healthy lifestyle information. Plus, they are tasked with some of the toughest challenges because lifestyle habits are so deeply ingrained in most of us.

The top five chronic disease killers today in modern societies don't just arise out of bad luck; they are largely the result of decades of unhealthy lifestyle choices and poor health habits, such as smoking, inactivity, managing stress poorly, and non-nutritious diets. We also know that socio-cultural conditions such as poverty, crime-ridden neighborhoods, racial and ethnic bias and discrimination, and structural violence all contribute to poor health and shorter longevity.

Health coaches are vitally important in an era when "diseases of lifestyle" account for almost 70 percent of the hospitalizations, physician visits and chronic illness today. Health and wellness coaches are trained in contemporary, evidence-based methods that support step-by-step change to reduce the risk of chronic disease, but more importantly, to partner with people so they can enjoy vibrant, active lives.

Integrative health coaches go one step further. They know that changing lifestyles is tough for most people, but there are soothing de-stressors and supportive therapies from the fields of integrative health and complementary medicine that provide extraordinary support as people try to overhaul their lifestyles while coping with a chronic condition. The emotional, physical, and financial cost of chronic health conditions can be devastating. The systems and techniques in this book have brought reliable relief to many people.

Integrative health coaches help people navigate the myriad of offerings in complementary, alternative, traditional, and holistic healing arts. The benefits of modalities such as herbs, massage, yoga, and acupuncture can vary from person to person. As complementary and alternative medicine (CAM) researcher, Jeanne Achterberg, PhD, once said, "Not every approach works for everybody; some things work for some bodies, and like all medicine, no one thing works all the time for everyone." Millions of people have been helped by various complementary approaches like targeted vitamin supplements or chiropractic care, but remain reluctant to talk with their regular medical doctors about them. A professionally-trained integrative health coach bridges the gap to provide support and facilitate communication with conventional healthcare providers. Wise consumer choices include a wide panoply of healing practitioners, including naturopathic medicine doctors, homeopaths, chiropractors, somatic therapists, and many more.

How to Use This Guide

Each graduate student researched and wrote about one specific modality or healing system. They followed this template: Definition, History, Philosophy, Treatments, What to Expect in a Session, Best Suited For, Contraindications, Research and Benefits, Practitioner Training and Credentials, Resources, and References. They also offered their own coaching tips.

How do you know if a certain modality or system is right for you as a coach or your client?

The primary issues of cost, access, and quality of service drive most of the decisions for individuals as they work with integrative health coaches. Is the complementary modality culturally appropriate and sensitive to the needs of families with diverse background? Is the modality supported in their neighborhood and conveniently located? Does the practice enjoy a wider acceptance and positive word-of-mouth? Do friends and neighbors talk about their successful outcomes? Does your doctor support the choice?

Sometimes people choose complementary or alternative paths because the conventional medical treatments have severe limitations or side effects. *Does* the alternative warrant a reconsideration since better outcomes are offered for less cost, less trouble? Is it legally available and are there consumer safeguards protecting the public? What is the assurance of safety and cost of care? Has a code of ethics been developed for this unconventional approach?

While all the above takes some time and effort to explore, each entry in this guide offers the following information to assist you. You will be able to:

- Find a simple definition and category featured at the top of each entry.

- Read the history and philosophy of each approach. Historical evidence of long-standing effective use in the human population should make you feel at ease.
- Learn how each modality or system is offered in terms of setting, duration and cost of typical treatments.
- Discover which chronic conditions are best treated by each modality or system.
- Be sure to read the list of contraindications.
- Inform yourself of the valid research and associated benefits.
- Learn what training and proper credentials are required or ideal for each of the practitioners and healing traditions.
- Rely on the resources and references that are offered.

It's still a buyer-beware marketplace for many complementary, alternative, and traditional healing arts, so take a proactive role in asking for recommendations and informing your regular healthcare providers about your intentions, choices, and experiences.

Finally, remember that there is a lot within your own scope of practice as a health coach that brings comfort and relief to people with chronic ailments. Introducing a calming breath technique or practice of mindfulness meditation is non-invasive, easy to learn, convenient, and effective. More than anything, this guide will help you expand your client's inner and outer resources, while you both learn how to evaluate options for increasing wellbeing.

INTEGRATIVE HEALTH:
A NEW PARADIGM FOR HEALTH AND HEALING
Meg Jordan

Today many organizations and leaders have adopted the term *integrative health*, rather than integrative medicine, since medicine implied the practice of medicine, exclusive to physicians, when the reality of integrative work encompasses a much broader field, including wellness managers, health coaches, psychotherapists, social workers, pastoral or spiritual teachers, fitness trainers, organic food chefs, recreational therapists, and more.

Integrative medicine is defined as the blending of complementary and alternative medicine (CAM) together with conventional or allopathic medicine, *complementary* being the modalities that harmonize easily with conventional medicine (vitamin therapy, massage, guided imagery), and *alternative* referring to those systems that have different etiological frameworks or worldviews (i.e., traditional Chinese medicine or Ayurvedic medicine). Integrative medicine is medicine that works, no matter if the source is conventional, complementary, or alternative.

Integrative health relies upon evidence-based, safe and effective medicines and healing approaches, along with valid principles of lifestyle or preventive medicine from a variety of traditions. As conventional medicine attempts to assist people with chronic ailments, it is often at its limit, if drugs or more invasive, costly interventions fail to produce desired results, or if patients cannot tolerate side effects. This is where integrative health can usher in more choices that may not all have the same level of scientific evidence but are useful in bringing about healthful outcomes. Generally, integrative health choices follow a continuum, starting with self-initiated care and behavior change, moving to the gentlest interventions, and finally, to the more invasive as a last resort.

The burgeoning field of integrative health draws fresh thinking and solutions from a world of healing options, including a broad understanding of complementary therapies such as naturopathic medicine, chiropractic, nutrition, diet and targeted supplementation, fitness and exercise, stress management, and yoga therapy, along with diverse, global healing approaches such as Ayurveda, traditional Chinese medicine, indigenous healing arts, and folk medicine. The cutting-edge approaches of functional medicine and personalized lifestyle medicine, coupled with genetic counseling, are also part of comprehensive integrative healthcare.

Just as wisdom traditions assure us that crisis gives rise to opportunity, the emergence of integrative health arrives as a healing balm for a costly and fragmented healthcare system in need of reform. However, integrative health seems to heal more than an ailing system, it also seems to heal the healers themselves, as epistemological divides are reconciled among CAM and conventionally educated practitioners. It is no wonder that integrative health continues to attract more clients as a preferred route of recovery from illness and relief from stressful lives. The out-of-pocket expenditures for integrative healthcare now exceeds that of mainstream medicine. The goal of CIIS Integrative Health Studies is to create leaders within healthcare that bring the principles and goals of integrative health to people everywhere, thereby transforming healthcare itself, and facilitating optimal wellbeing for self and others.

What About Evidence?

A common, and rather invalid, criticism directed toward integrative and complementary health practices is that they lack sufficient evidence—a statement that more accurately points to a lack of clarity about what *evidence* really means. There are many levels of evidence, from long-term historical usage indicating general safety, to observational pilot studies, to more rigorous case reports, to well-designed clinical studies, and finally, the randomized, double-blind clinical trial and meta-analysis of several trials.

What few people realize is that less than half of conventional medicine's treatments are evidence based. The vast majority of medical practice is based on trial-and-error observations, consensus-built protocols and no small amount of experimentation. Likewise, not everything in a complementary modality such as herbalism should be accepted because it is deemed "natural" or nature-based. The test for safety was traditionally earned through centuries of historical usage, until more recent clinical trials mounted increasing evidence of the validity of many complementary and alternative healing remedies.

The following **Six Principles of Integrative Health** are taught within the CIIS Integrative Health Studies M.A. program.

1. Integrative health rests on a foundation of a unified whole (*hale,* original Latin for wholeness or health).

    Mind is restored to body; spirit to matter; and subjective, without objective ways of knowing, are acknowledged and valued. Integrative health practitioners combine ancient wisdom with modern science, modalities from around the world, and individual responsibility within cultural support.

2. Integrative health requires respectful collaboration among multiple disciplines.

    Integrative health practitioners restore a time-honored canon of supportive therapeutic relationships, deep levels of collaboration with other practitioners. Research by faculty at the CIIS M.A.

program involves multidisciplinary healing circles that benefit persons with long-standing chronic ailments.

3. Integrative health is relationship-centered and holds the client to be ultimately resourceful, whole and having a narrative that is central to healing.

    The clients' narratives inspire a commitment among integrative health practitioners to keep client needs and preferences central and directive to their process of healing and recovery. Shared decision-making and co-created wellness visions are products of keeping the client at the center of the healing journey.

4. Integrative health seeks to restore the dynamic balance of a living system.

    Dynamic balance is the fluid state of the self-organizing, self-correcting processes within the micro/macrocellular, biochemical, neuroendocrine, musculoskeletal, and hemodynamic systems of the body interacting with its environment. Integrative health honors the intrinsic healing capacity within all living organisms, and acknowledges how that capacity requires interpersonal, societal, and ecological cooperation and wellbeing.

5. Integrative health is preventive, proactive, effective, and efficient.

    Integrative health seeks to accomplish the "triple aim" of the National Academies of Science, Engineering and Medicine: quality improvement, cost containment, and improved health outcomes within healthcare systems. Practitioners are able to refer to reliable sources of information and seek first to do the least invasive, least costly form of intervention. Since the original conception of Triple Aim, a Fourth Aim has been added: care and support for the healers themselves, an urgently needed addition to counter rising rates of stress, burnout, and even suicide for doctors, nurses and other helping professionals. Integrative health should permeate all the corridors of conventional healthcare.

6. Integrative health honors health equity.

    Integrative health is built on a foundation of advocacy for multicultural perspectives, cultural sensitivity, social justice and health equity. Core values include fair access, empowered decision-making, client-centered care, and affordability. These values are upheld by integrative health practitioners.

ACUPRESSURE
Cynthia Espinoza

Where there is no movement there is pain. Where there is movement there is no pain.

—Traditional Chinese axiom

Acupressure is a modality known to traditional Chinese medicine. The modality involves a practitioner pressing on the pressure points of the body with their hands or with massage tools. The pressure is believed to restore health by alleviating mental, emotional, or physical discomfort (Yifang, 9). Practitioners report that the flow of *qi,* or vital energy, is restored because functional imbalances or blocks are released by stimulating these pressure points along the body's meridians. This treatment does not involve puncturing the body as in acupuncture (McFadden & Hernández, 2010). Overall, the use of this pressure strives to bring balance back to the body.

History
Acupressure was developed in ancient China over 5,000 years ago (Wren & Norred, 179). During early Asian empires, soldiers in battle noticed that they experienced relief from other physical ailments after being hit with rocks and arrows. Although they were struck in various areas of the body, they later noticed other seemingly unrelated health issues resolved themselves. This recovery was a shock to doctors who did not know how to connect the instances. Through continued tests and tribulations, doctors created acupressure (Gach, 4).

Acupressure has been practiced as a folk art that has made its way through generations. Along with its presence in China, acupressure has recorded practice in Japan and India (Gach, 6). While the technique has been practiced in many places over time, the purpose of acupressure remains the same among the people who practice it. All participants want to manifest and maintain free flowing energy in the human body (Gach, 12).

Since 1991, there has been an increased use of acupressure in the US, when the Office of Alternative Medicine (OAM) was established at the National Institutes of Health (NIH), now called the National Center for Complementary and Integrative Health. As research accumulated on the benefits of traditional Chinese medicine, both acupressure and acupuncture underwent a rise in interest and usage.

Philosophy

Acupressure is utilized as a technique that promotes the flow of "chi" or "qi," which is known as a vital source of energy that brings life and health to the body (Micozzi, 129). Chi runs through energy pathways known as meridians. These meridians are associated with different organs. It is believed that illnesses and ailments block the free movement of chi (Mehta, 251). Therefore, acupressure is thought to help unblock meridians so that chi can resume carrying energy for us to feel healthy and lively again (Micozzi, 129).

In addition, acupressure works to balance the universal yin and yang forces. Yin is believed to represent a calm, passive, and bright force. Yang represents a darker, physical, and energetic force. The dominance of one or the other may fluctuate during times of difficulty or the seasons. Yin is associated with the internal body and yang correlates with the exterior skin. When pressure is placed on the body during an acupressure treatment, yin and yang are thought to produce energy because the treatment merges the two opposing parts (Luckmann, 201). Having them equally in play makes for a more stable level of health (Dalet, 14).

Treatments: What to Expect

Acupressure addresses the same 365 pressure points that are used in acupuncture therapy (Stillerman, 1). There are multiple styles of acupressure, each of which is unique in the way that it addresses each pressure point and the length of pressure applied. Each style uses of pressure points differently and can use more than the typical 365 points. The many styles include shiatsu, jin shin jyutsu, tui na, tsubo, Watsu, and ohashiatsu (Snyder & Lindquist, 256; Wren & Norred, 180). A session involves the use of thumbs, fingers, and/or knuckles to open up these energy pathways (Stillerman, 1). There are also bracelets, spoons, and other massage tools that are designated for the use of acupressure.

An effective acupressure session may leave you feeling a bit sore, but not in pain. The soreness may feel light to moderate and should feel more like it is positively helping you heal (Stillerman, 3). The soreness is brought on by the release of lactic acid and toxins in the body.

Setting: Self-administered wherever comfortable, or professional's office.
Duration: 45–90 minutes.
Cost: $65–110.

Best Suited for These Conditions

- Allergies
- Stress
- Anxiety
- Depression
- Back/neck pain
- Lethargy
- Digestive issues or disorders
- Menstrual cramps
- Discomfort during childbirth
- Headache
- Nausea
- Trouble sleeping
- Fibromyalgia

Coaching Tip

A noninvasive alternative to acupuncture, acupressure addresses a wide array of ailments ranging from emotional to physical wellbeing. You may find that clients who appreciate therapeutic massage but are unfamiliar with traditional Chinese medicine are curious about the benefits of acupressure.

Contraindications

- Acupressure should be avoided if clients have:
- Infection
- Skin disease
- Open wounds, burns, swelling, or ulcers on or near a meridian
- Recently done rigorous exercise or movement
- Full stomach
- Tuberculosis
- Stomach cancer
- Leukemia
- Serious cardiac dysfunction
- Pregnancy (if done incorrectly, acupressure may cause premature birth)

Research and Benefits

The benefits that an individual can gain from acupressure treatment are contingent upon how often the client interacts with the treatment. After one session, results can last up to two or three days. However, with more

Integrative Health Coaching

consistent practice, acupressure can leave individuals with lifelong rewards (Stillerman, 2).

Scientists have researched and tried to reason why acupressure works for some individuals. They have found that through pressure, the body may produce electromagnetic signals that promote the circulation of pain-killing biochemicals, like that of endorphins (Wren & Norred, 179). In addition, acupressure may stimulate immune system cells to migrate to places of injury or sickness in the body. Further, acupressure may also reduce pain and discomfort by triggering the body's opiate system.

When the body goes through prolonged periods of stress, injury, physiological imbalance, disease, or lack of diet or movement, the body's muscles tighten around acupressure points due to the secretion of lactic acid (Gach, 5). However, the overall ease of muscle tension may also be the result of the release of lactic acid through the physical contact produced in acupressure (Wren and Norred, 179).

Among a few studies that have been performed, acupressure has been used with patients going through chemotherapy (Dibble et al., 813), post-stroke rehabilitation (McFadden and Hernández, 1), or childbirth labor pains (Lee, 959). These studies have all found positive results in easing discomfort from nausea, vomiting, and pain, and have found that acupressure increases relaxation.

Practitioner Training and Credentials
There is no specified credential solely for administering acupressure. Practitioners usually hold a license or certification in massage therapy, nursing, or acupuncture (DrWeil.com). From there, practitioners can get extra training to become specialized in acupressure. The American Oriental Bodywork Therapy Association has created the standards for treatment that practitioners must then abide by (Wren & Norred, 182). As people continue to seek and learn more about alternative therapies, they have become more interested in learning about acupressure so that they can apply it to themselves (Bauer, 5). Self-applied acupressure is convenient because it is simple, cost effective, and easy to learn (Bauer, 4).

Resources
Informative acupressure website—acupressure.com
Search for local acupressure practitioner—thumbtack.com
Acuhealth's acupressure guide—acuhealth.com.au/body.html
Acupressure for beginners—exploreim.ucla.edu/self-care/acupressure-and-
    common-acupressure-points

References

"Acupressure—Dr. Weil's Wellness Therapies."—DrWeil.com. drweil.com/health-wellness/balanced-living/wellness-therapies/acupressure. Accessed May 2017.

Bauer, C. *Acupressure for Women*. Crossing Press, 1987.

Beal, MW. "Acupuncture and Acupressure." *Journal of Nurse-Midwifery* 44, no.3 (1999). 217–230. doi: 10.1016/S0091-2182(99)00054-3

Dalet, R. *How to Give Yourself Relief from Pain by the Simple Pressure of a Finger*. Stein and Day, 1982.

Dibble, SL, et al. "Acupressure for Chemotherapy-Induced Nausea and Vomiting: A Randomized Clinical Trial." *Oncology Nursing Forum* 34, no. 4 (2007).

Gach, MR. *Basic Acupressure: the Extraordinary Channels & Points*. Acupressure.com, 2008.

"Health Costs." How Much Does Acupressure Cost? 2017. howmuchisit.org/acupressure-cost.

Hsieh, LL, et al. "A Randomized Controlled Clinical Trial for Low Back Pain Treated by Acupressure and Physical Therapy." *Preventive Medicine*, 39, no. 1 (July 2004).168–176.

Lee, MK, Chang, SB, & Kang, D-H. "Effects of SP6 Acupressure on Labor Pain and Length of Delivery Time in Women During Labor." *The Journal of Alternative and Complementary Medicine* 10, no. 6 (2004). 959–965.

Luckmann, W. "Daoist Pain Management: Balancing Acupressure Technique." *Massage & Bodywork* 25, no. 4 (Jul/Aug 2010). 68–77.

McFadden, KL, & Hernández, TD. "Cardiovascular Benefits of Acupressure (Jin Shin) Following Stroke." *Complementary Therapies in Medicine* 18 no.1 (2010). 42–48.

Mehta, P, Dhapte, V, Kadam, S, & Dhapte, V. "Contemporary acupressure therapy: Adroit cure for painless recovery of therapeutic ailments." *Journal of Traditional and Complementary Medicine* 7, no. 2 (2017). 251–63. sciencedirect.com/science/article/pii/S222541101630044X.

Micozzi, MS. *Fundamentals of Complementary and Integrative Medicine*. 3rd ed. Saunders Elsevier, 2006.

Pinzón-Pérez, H, & Pérez, MA. "Chapter 4: Manipulative and Body-Based Practices." *Complementary, Alternative, and Integrative Health: A Multicultural Perspective*. Jossey-Bass & Pfeiffer Imprints, Wiley, 2016. 98–101.

Snyder, M, Lindquist, R, & Weiss, P. "Chapter 20: Acupressure." *Complementary/Alternative Therapies in Nursing*. 5th ed. Springer Publishing , 2006. 255–69.

Stillerman, E. *Encyclopedia of Bodywork: From Acupressure to Zone Therapy.* Facts On File, 1996.

Wren, KR & Norred, CL. "Section 5: Healing With Subtle Energy-Acupressure." *Real World Nursing Survival Guide: Complementary and Alternative Therapies.* Saunders, 2003: 179–182.

Wu, B. Effect of acupuncture on the regulation of cell-mediated immunity in the patients with malignant tumors. *Chen Tzu Yen Chiu Acupuncture Research* 20, no. 3(1995). 67–71.

Wu, B, Zhou, RX, & Zhou, MS. "Effect of acupuncture on interleukin-2 level and NK cell immunoactivity of peripheral blood of malignant tumor patients." *Chung Kuo Chung Hsi I Chieh Ho Tsa Chich (Chin J Mod Dev Trad Med)* 14, no. 9 (1994). 537–539.

Yifang, Z. *Using Traditional Chinese Medicine to Manage your Emotional Health: How Herbs, Natural Foods, and Acupressure Can Regulate and Harmonize your Mind and Body.* Better Link, 2013.

ACUPUNCTURE
Laura Katz

Originating in China, acupuncture is an ancient system of healing that inserts and stimulates hair-thin needles at various sites along the body's energy lines (meridians) to unblock the flow of energy and restore balance and health.

History

Acupuncture was first documented as a cohesive system of diagnosis and treatment in *The Yellow Emperor's Classic of Internal Medicine*, around 100 BCE. Acupuncture continued to develop over the centuries and gradually became one of the standard therapies used in China, along with herbs, massage, diet and moxibustion (heat). During the Ming Dynasty (1368-1644), *The Great Compendium of Acupuncture and Moxibustion* was published—the text that forms the basis of modern acupuncture. (The Long History of Chinese Medicine-Briefly) Acupuncture spread to other countries at various times, by different routes. Differing acupuncture traditions such as Japanese and Korean ones use notably different techniques than Chinese acupuncture, however the basic theoretical premise is the same. (Maciocia) Divergent strands of acupuncture were brought together under Chairman Mao in the 1950s in communist China, in part to provide healthcare to China's large population. In 1972, with the founding of the first US acupuncture organization, the education of Chinese medicine expanded to include Western doctors and dentists (The Long History of Chinese Medicine-Briefly). Acupuncture grew to be more accepted in the US in 1997 when the National Institutes of Health reported positive evidence for its effectiveness, at least in a limited range of conditions (Marwick, 1725). Acupuncture is now recognized as a therapeutic modality in the US, and treatment is often covered by health insurance.

Philosophy

Traditional Chinese medicine theorizes that more than 2,000 acupuncture points on the human body connect with twelve main and eight secondary pathways called meridians. These meridians conduct energy, or qi, between the surface of the body and internal organs. Qi regulates spiritual, emotional, mental, and physical balance. Qi is influenced by the opposing forces of yin and yang. When yin and yang are balanced, they work together with the natural flow of qi to help the body achieve and maintain health. Acupuncture is believed to balance yin and yang, keep the normal flow of energy unblocked, and restore health to the body and mind.

Disease is viewed as an energy imbalance or stagnation. Acupuncture stimulates energy meridians in order to reestablish balance and allow stagnated energy to flow to restore harmony to the body (American Academy of Medical Acupuncture). Along with the theory of yin and yang, the theory of the five elements forms the basis of Chinese medicine and acupuncture. The five elements in nature are water, fire, wood, metal, and earth. These five elements correspond to organs and qi in the body. (Maciocia)

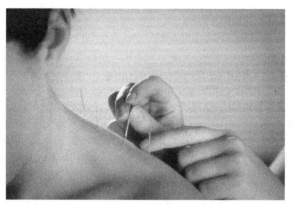

Treatments: What to Expect

The first visit involves a thorough exam and interview during which the acupuncturist assesses the patient's health needs and energy imbalances. During this assessment the acupuncturist performs a Chinese pulse diagnosis and evaluates the tongue, hair, nails, complexion, and more. The acupuncturist also asks questions related to aspects of daily life, such as sleep patterns and appetite. Acupuncturists often make lifestyle and dietary recommendations, as they hold a holistic view of health and wellness.

Overall the experience is pleasant for most people. The patient may experience some sensation upon the insertion of the sterile, hair-thin needle. This pinch or pressure at the moment of insertion quickly subsides. Often patients experience an energetic flow from the point of insertion to some part of the body, followed by deep relaxation. Many patients fall asleep during treatment. The calm, clear-headed sensation lasts for some time after treatment, depending on the patient. Treatment experiences vary among patients, and often vary from treatment to treatment for the same person. Even if there are no sensations, a treatment can be quite beneficial. At the end of treatment, the needles are removed and discarded.

Setting: Private room. Community acupuncture can be administered to multiple patients.

Duration: 30–60 minutes.

Cost: $80–150 for private session, $15–60 for community session.

Best Suited for These Conditions

- Anxiety
- Arthritis
- Asthma
- Bronchitis
- Carpal tunnel syndrome
- Chronic fatigue
- Common cold
- Depression
- Digestive trouble
- Fatigue
- Fibromyalgia
- Headache
- Insomnia/sleep disturbances
- Irritable bowel syndrome
- Menopause
- Menstrual irregularities
- Migraine
- Morning sickness
- Nausea
- Osteoarthritis
- Pain: neck, back, shoulder, knee, etc.
- Plantar fasciitis
- PMS
- Reproductive problems/fertility
- Sciatica
- Sinusitis
- Smoking cessation
- Stress management
- Urinary tract infections

Coaching Tip

It is easy to tailor your recommendation for acupuncture to your client. If your client is open to discussing energy fields, chi, meridians, etc., then use that in your discussion. However, if your client is used to Western-style medicine, acupuncture has been widely studied, applied and accepted in Western medicine. It is often covered by health insurance and you can discuss acupuncture studies without ever speaking of qi, or the subtle energy body, if necessary, to meet your client's needs. Acupuncture is gentle, holistic, and has virtually no side effects.

Contraindications

The patient must be able to hold still long enough for treatment, but a skilled acupuncturist can work with most patients. Even animals such as dogs, cats, and horses can receive acupuncture with great benefit. Some patients may not be good candidates because of a significant fear of needles.

Practitioner Training and Credentials

Each state requires a license, certification, or registration to practice acupuncture, although educational requirements and training standards vary among states. A license indicates that the practitioner meets certain standards regarding the knowledge and use of acupuncture.

Resources

Accreditation Commission for Acupuncture and Oriental Medicine (ACAOM)
7501 Greenway Center Drive, Suite 820
Greenbelt, MD 20770
(301) 313-0855
acaom.org

Acupuncture and Oriental Medicine National Coalition
750 East Sample Road (2-209)
Pompano Beach, FL 33064
(954) 494-2903
info@aomnc.comaomnc.com

American Academy of Medical Acupuncture (AAMA)
5820 Wilshire Boulevard, Suite 500
Los Angeles, CA 90036
(323) 937-5514
medicalacupuncture.org

American Academy of Veterinary Acupuncture
P.O. Box 419
Hygiene, CO 80533-0419
(303) 772-6726
AAVAoffice@aol.com aava.org

American Association of Acupuncture and Oriental Medicine (AAAOM)
P.O. Box 96503, #44114,
Washington DC 20090-6503
866-455-7999
awoodward@aaaomonline.org   aaaomonline.org

National Acupuncture Foundation (NAF)
P.O. Box 2271
Gig Harbor, WA 98335-4271
(253) 851-6538

National Certification Commission for Acupuncture and Oriental Medicine (NCCAOM)
76 Laurel Street, Suite 1290
Jacksonville, FL 32202
(703) 548-9004
nccaom.org

References

"Acupuncture: In Depth." *National Center for Complementary and Integrative Health*, US Department of Health and Human Services, 21 Feb. 2017, nccih.nih.gov/health/acupuncture/introduction#hed2.

"American Academy of Medical Acupuncture " *American Academy of Medical Acupuncture*. medicalacupuncture.org.

American Association of Acupuncture and Oriental Medicine. aaaomonline.org/Patients.

"The Long History of Chinese Medicine-Briefly." *American College of Traditional Chinese Medicine*, 8 July 2015. actcm.edu/news/stories/the-long-history-of-chinese-medicine-briefly.

Maciocia, G. *The Foundations of Chinese Medicine: a Comprehensive Text for Acupuncturists and Herbalists*. Elsevier Churchill Livingstone, 2006.

Marwick, C. "Acceptance of Some Acupuncture Applications." *JAMA* 278, no. 21 (1997). 1725. doi: 10.1001/jama.1997.03550210021013.

White, A. "A Brief History of Acupuncture." *Rheumatology* 43, no. 5 (2004). 662–663. doi: 10.1093/rheumatology/keg005.

AROMATHERAPY
Marissa Poulin

Aromatherapy is the practice of using concentrated essential oils extracted from volatile plant materials to enhance psychological and physical wellbeing as part of a holistic treatment approach.

History

Aromatherapy and essential oils have been used as natural remedies by ancient cultures worldwide for thousands of years. It is believed that the ancient Egyptians invented the first rudimentary distillation equipment and used oils infused with herbs for rituals, embalming, medicine, cosmetics, and perfume (Aromatherapy, A Brief History). In the 19th century, scientists analyzed the medicinal uses of essential oils and documented their findings. Aromatherapy was used by nurses in hospitals as a way to reduce the amount of pain and anxiety their patients were experiencing, as well as to increase their wellbeing, and to provide additional therapeutic support to the healing process (The Center for Health & Healing).

The term *aromatherapy* was first used in 1910 by René-Maurice Gattefossé, a French chemist who experienced a bad burn while working in his laboratory and plunged his arm into the nearest vat of liquid, which was filled with lavender oil. He was amazed that the burn healed so quickly and didn't scar, which further piqued his interest in essential oils. He studied both the psychological and physiological effects of essential oils and first used the word aromatherapy in his 1937 publication *Aromathérapie: Les Huiles essentielles hormones végétales* (The Center for Health & Healing).

Other significant people who helped pave the way for the modern practice of aromatherapy include Jean Valnet, who used eucalyptus as a bactericide to treat wounded soldiers during WWII; Madame Marguerite Maury, an Austrian biochemist who introduced aromatherapy into cosmetics and massage; and Robert B. Tisserand, an English aromatherapist who brought aromatherapy to English-speaking populations and wrote the first aromatherapy book published in English in 1977, *The Art of Aromatherapy* (Aromatherapy, A Brief History).

Philosophy

Aromatherapy uses natural essential oils found in plants; the oils are extracted either by steam distillation or expression. Steam distillation is the method used most prominently and involves steaming the plant matter until it breaks down into the fragrant oil. This oil is then cooled, separated from the water, and filtered into its pure essential oil. The expression method involves pressing the plant to extract the oils (Aromatherapy—The Balance & Harmony of Body and Mind, 2010).

Essential oils are powerful aromatic compounds found in plants that help protect them from disease and insects and make them more attractive to pollinators. Likewise, these oils offer humans natural remedies to prevent and treat ailments. There are complex chemical components found in essential oils that have medicinal properties and can affect the mind and body in a variety of ways. These oils can be administered by inhalation or massage, or in lotions, compresses, and steam baths. The synergy of different essential oils is an important element when considering using aromatherapy as a therapeutic tool. Blending oils can have a more powerful effect than using just one oil alone.

There are numerous physical and psychological benefits of using aromatherapy, including its ability to relieve stress, decrease feelings of depression and anxiety, reduce pain, increase energy levels, increase rates of healing and recovery, improve memory, regulate sleep, reduce headaches and migraines, bolster the immune system, and improve digestion. Essential oils also have antibacterial, anti-inflammatory, antiseptic, and analgesic properties when used topically (Althea Press).

Practitioners believe that the beneficial effects of aromatherapy result from chemical molecules in the essential oils binding to olfactory receptors, which sends impulses to the limbic system, the part of the brain that regulates emotions and memories. Depending on which oil is used, there may be a calming or stimulating effect on the body.

Treatments: What to Expect

Aromatherapy oils can be used in a variety of ways. One mode of application is to inhale the essential oil vapors directly, or to add a few drops of oil to steaming water, bathwater, diffusers, or candles. The aroma will activate the olfactory sense, which will improve circulation and help to evoke a sense of wellbeing. Topical application of essential oils can be administered by blending a few drops to massage oils, lotions, or salves, or by applying warm compresses directly to areas needing pain relief. The oils are absorbed directly into the skin and the bloodstream and generate beneficial healing effects. It is not recommended that pure essential oils be applied directly to the skin because they are highly concentrated and may cause irritation.

Setting: Professional setting or at home.

Duration: No set duration for using essential oils.

Cost: $5–100, depending on the quality and brand.

Best Suited for These Conditions

- Stress relief
- Anxiety
- Depression
- Pain in muscles, nerves, joints (arthritis), earache, and eyestrain
- Skin issues such as dermatitis, pimples, dry skin, burns, cuts, insect bites, poison ivy, warts, herpes, hives, athlete's foot, and varicose veins
- Fatigue
- Weak immune system
- Digestive issues
- Insomnia/trouble sleeping
- Impaired memory and Alzheimer's
- Headaches and migraines
- Menopause and PMS
- Poor circulation

Coaching Tip

If your client would like to see an aromatherapist, you might recommend that they ask for a personal recommendation from a doctor or friend, or search for one using the Aromatherapy Registration Council website. If your client is interested in using essential oils at home, recommend that they choose quality oils from reputable brands such as doTERRA Essential Oils, Plant Therapy Essential Oils, or Young Living Essential Oils. Caution them to research the safest way to use essential oils.

Contraindications

It is important for aromatherapy practitioners to understand both the uses of essential oils and their toxicities, side effects, and possible interactions with medications. It is important to note is that pure essential oils should never be directly applied to the skin; essential oils should always be diluted in a carrier oil, like coconut or olive oil. There can be possible side-effects from using a concentration that is too strong. "The potency of steam-distilled essential oils is up to 1000 times stronger than in the naturally occurring living plant. Because of this, the essential oil must be diluted in a carrier oil before use at a dilution ranging from .05% to 5%" (The Center for Health and Healing, 2012).

Vulnerable populations: Babies, elderly, and pregnant or breastfeeding women should avoid using certain essential oils because they tend to be more sensitive to them.

Toxicity: Ingestion of certain essential oils, such as mugwort, wintergreen, and eucalyptus, can be toxic and may cause damage to the nervous system, liver, and kidneys.

Skin irritation: When applied to the skin in undiluted form, certain essential oils can cause rashes, itching, and burning sensations, depending on the person's sensitivity or allergies.

Photosensitivity: Oils like cumin, lemon, bergamot, and angelica root can cause sunburn when they are applied to skin that will be exposed to the sun for long periods of time.

Reaction with medications: Some oils (ingested or topical) can potentially have negative interactions with medicines. The best way to ensure a positive experience with essential oils is to communicate with your doctor about your intended use for the oils.

Research and Benefits

Relieve Stress: Stress relief is the most common use for aromatherapy. Some of the essential oils that act as relaxants that can help calm the mind and reduce anxious feelings include lavender, lemon oil, peppermint, bergamot, and ylang-ylang.

Reduce Depression: Aromatherapy can be used to elevate mood and alleviate symptoms of depression, as well as improve physical and mental wellbeing. Aromas from essential oils are carried directly to the limbic system, which controls emotional responses like depression, anger, and fear. Essential oils such as bergamot, chamomile, sandalwood, lavender, peppermint, and jasmine are great for boosting mood and lowering feelings of depression.

Improve Memory: Many people use aromatherapy as a complementary treatment for memory-related diseases such as dementia and Alzheimer's. One study showed that patients with Alzheimer's disease showed significant improvement in cognitive function after using aromatherapy oils like rosemary, lemon, lavender, and orange for a 28-day period (Jimbo, Daiki et al.). Studies have also shown sage oil to boost memory capacity of younger patients (10 Amazing Benefits of Aromatherapy).

Boost Energy: Essential oils like lemon, ginger, peppermint, black pepper, grapefruit, angelica, rosemary, and basil can help increase circulation and stimulate the body and mind, and therefore boost energy levels.

Speed up Healing: Many essential oils can help stimulate the healing process by increasing oxygen and blood flow to wounds. The antimicrobial and antibacterial properties of certain essential oils also protect the body during the healing process. The best essential oils for speeding up the healing process include clove, eucalyptus, lavender, oregano, tea tree, rose hip, and peppermint.

Relieve Headaches and Migraines: Essential oils like peppermint, eucalyptus, lavender, and rosemary help relieve headaches and migraines by minimizing the triggers that cause them, such as stress, tension, and sinus pressure. These oils can also be used with a carrier oil and massaged onto the temples, back of neck, and scalp.

Sleep Aid: Essential oils can be diffused to create a calming and peaceful environment in the bedroom, which is favorable for sleeping. Essential oils that are great for improving sleep include lavender, sweet marjoram, chamomile, sandalwood, jasmine, and ylang-ylang. "[These oils] can also be used topically and taken internally to calm the nervous system, promote relaxation, and lead to a restful sleep" (6 Tips for A Better Night's Sleep).

Boost Immune System: Certain essential oils have antimicrobial, antibacterial, and antifungal properties that can help ward off illnesses and infections that could cause damage to the body's systems. Immunity-boosting oils include cinnamon, lemon, oregano, peppermint, frankincense, and eucalyptus.

Pain Relief: Aromatherapy can be used to soothe tense muscles, achy joints, and inflammation. The best essential oils for pain relief include lavender, chamomile, juniper, eucalyptus, rosemary, and peppermint.

Improve Digestion: Aromatherapy can help alleviate bloating, gas, constipation, indigestion, and increase metabolism. The best essential oils for treating digestive conditions are citrus oils, like lemon and orange.

Practitioner Training and Credentials

Aromatherapy is currently an unregulated field, and there is no official aromatherapy accreditation in the US. People wishing to become aromatherapists can obtain a certificate from a number of schools or organizations that provide online training. A certification from an aromatherapy school is not a national certification nor is it a license to practice; it simply means that the criteria required by that organization were met. Many alternative healthcare practitioners, such as massage therapists, aestheticians, naturopaths, energy healers, and Ayurvedic clinicians, utilize their aromatherapy certificates to complement their existing practice. There are also people who obtain a certificate in aromatherapy because they have a passion for natural healing and want to learn more about this therapy and to help others.

Most aromatherapy programs are online or weekend workshops, and the number of required training hours varies anywhere from 10–300 hours. There are also a few programs that are geared towards healthcare practitioners, which require the student to either already have a degree or license in their field of expertise or be enrolled in an approved college. Prices can range $50–2,000, depending on the organization (Aromatherapy Courses).

Aromatherapy is currently overseen by several trade associations, the National Association for Holistic Aromatherapy (NAHA), Natural Oils Research Association (NORA), Alliance of International Aromatherapists (AIA), and Aromatherapy Registration Council (ARC). The accreditation goals of these organizations include setting educational standards, fostering ethics and integrity in the education and practice of aromatherapy across the community, creating guidelines for the safe use of oils, educating about sustainability issues in aromatherapy, and upholding other professional requirements to obtain and keep certification as an aromatherapist (Aromatherapy Courses). These organizations also serve to connect practitioners and community members, as well as raise awareness about aromatherapy to the public.

Resources
General information about Aromatherapy—aromatherapy.com
National Association for Holistic Aromatherapy—naha.org
Alliance of International Aromatherapists—alliance-aromatherapists.org
Aromatherapy Registration Council—aromatherapycouncil.org

References
"6 Tips for a Better Night's Sleep | Doterra Essential Oils." *Doterra.com*, 2017, doterra.com/US/en/blog/healthy-living-sleep-what-many-of-us-are-missing. Accessed 6 April, 2017.

"10 Amazing Benefits of Aromatherapy | Organic Facts." Organic Facts, 2017, organicfacts.net/health-benefits/other/benefits-of-aromatherapy.html. Accessed 2 April, 2017.

Althea Press. *Essential Oils Natural Remedies*. Althea Press, 2015.

"Aromatherapy, A Brief History" Edenbotanicals.com, 2012, edenbotanicals.com/aromatherapy-a-brief-history. Accessed 29 March, 2017.

"Aromatherapy Courses | Aromatherapy Training and Licensure." Natural Healers, 2017, naturalhealers.com/alternative-medicine/aromatherapy-career. Accessed 29 March, 2017.

"Aromatherapy—The Balance & Harmony of Body and Mind" Aromatherapy.com, 2010, aromatherapy.com/essential_oils.html. Accessed 2 April, 2017.

Jimbo, D, et al. "Effect of Aromatherapy on Patients with Alzheimer's Disease." *Psychogeriatrics* 9, no. 4 (2009): 173–179. doi: 10.1111/j.1479-8301.2009.00299.x.

"The Center for Health & Healing." Healthandhealingny.com, 2012, healthandhealingny.com/complement/aroma_history.html. Accessed 4 April, 2017.

AYURVEDA
Ana Benuelas Balderas

Ayurveda, the "science of life," is a mind-body health system created in India approximately 5,000 years ago.

History and Philosophy

Ayurveda is a word derived from ancient roots—*ayus* (life) and *ved* (knowledge). Ayurveda is more than a health system designed to treat illness. It is a science of life created to help people maintain balanced and healthy human potential. Following an Ayurvedic practice will help you toward optimal health.

Ayurveda has two main guiding principles: the body and the mind are inextricably connected, and there is nothing more powerful to heal and transform the body than the mind (Chopra). In order to develop freedom from illness, it is important to cultivate an awareness practice and then extend that mindfulness to the rest of the body. You can achieve a calm mind and state of awareness through the practice of meditation.

There are different aspects to learn in order to build a stronger Ayurvedic practice. First, you must know your mind-body type. These are outlined in the table.

	Vata Movement and change	Pitta Transformation and metabolism	Kapha Structure and fluidity
Elements	Space and air	Fire and water	Water and earth
Qualities	Cold, light, dry, changeable, and moving.	Hot, light, intense, acidic, and pungent.	Heavy, slow, soft, cold, and oily.
Body type	Thin and agile. Light sleep and sensitive digestion.	Medium size and weight. Baldness, great digestion, short and noisy sleep.	Perfect stamina and strong build. Vibrant skin, thick hair, smooth, and constant digestion.

	Loves trying new things, being excited, and holding deep conversations.	Is intellectual, focused, and good speaker.	Is generally calm, loving, and thoughtful. Routine-friendly and enjoy life.
Character-istics			
In balance	Energetic, creative, and flexible.	Great energy, strong appetite, and ideal digestion.	Loyal, strong, patient, and supportive.

The Ayurveda system was created with the purpose of connecting with inner intelligence, of finding balance, and then bringing balance to the body. In this system, it is believed that the mind has the power to influence the path of our body into either health or sickness. Ayurveda has seven basic guiding principles created in order to help people restore and maintain that mind-body balance:

- Eat a healthy, colorful diet
- Sleep well at night
- Engage in regular exercise that promotes strength and flexibility
- Take daily time to meditate
- Cultivate loving and nurturing relationships
- End what does not serve you
- Awaken your passion

When you follow the Ayurveda lifestyle, you eventually create a better energy flow, which begins with your digestive system. Following the right diet for your body, you will eat the right amount you need in order to perform daily activities, and your body will not store anything it does not need. By doing so, you will be improving your immune system, nervous system, and circulatory system, in addition to finding emotional stability. You will also lose or gain weight in a healthy way, while keeping your body nourished.

Ayurveda accomplishes these goals by reducing *ama* while strengthening *agni*. Ama refers to the accumulated toxicity in the body, while agni is the Hindi term for fire. When the agni levels are low, the digestive system does not work at its peak, which results in the generation of ama or toxins in the body. In Ayurveda, it is believed that when your agni is deep and strong, it has the power to digest any kind of food and use it in keeping with your needs.

Treatments: What to Expect

A typical visit to an Ayurvedic practitioner will consist of an examination of your body; a personal and medical history; a discussion of the environment in which you live; and a review of your eating and exercise habits, your relationships, and other wellness areas. The practitioner will try to identify patterns and key factors that could be affecting your balance.

These are some of the common steps employed by Ayurvedic practitioners:

- Observation and evaluation of physical health in general
- Touch, such as tapping
- Laboratory testing
- Questions related to symptoms and complaints
- Individualized examination; Ayurvedic diagnosis is focused on the patient's component of the condition (rogi)
- Holistic considerations, including the energy factor your body may need to bring it back to balance
- Determination of your *dosha*, which is essential in order to identify the root cause of disease and find balance

Herbs and herbal formulas

The effects and effectiveness of each herb depends on its taste (*ras*), its active potency (*virya*), and its post-digestive effect (*vipak*). Ayurvedic herbs must be prescribed only by practitioners. Herbs are not necessarily benign and could have side effects, which is why a good knowledge and understanding of plants and herbs and its potential effects (physiological, biochemical, and psychological) are required.

Panchakarma

This Ayurvedic approach was created in order to promote detoxification by the removal of *ama* (toxins). The treatment can consist of several different approaches, from massage therapy to enemas.

Nutrition and Diet

Six tastes are sought for good health:

- Sweet: nourishes the tissues and promotes strength
- Sour: stimulates digestive power
- Salty: helps to maintain electrolyte balance
- Pungent: builds stronger digestion and absorption
- Bitter: stimulates all the other tastes
- Astringent: aids with optimal absorption

Ayurvedic Massage

Massage treatments are performed by trained therapists who should be working under the supervision of Ayurvedic practitioners. Ayurvedic massages are usually individualized and specific oils are selected according to the diagnosis made by the practitioner.

Shirodhara

A fine stream of hot liquid is poured over the forehead, which is believed to have healing effects related to the eyes, nose, head, neck, and the nervous system.

Setting: Professional office.
Duration: Varies depending on work-up and type of treatment.
Cost: $70-200.

Best Suited for These Conditions

- Ayurvedic practices have been shown to be helpful for treating hormonal, inflammatory, digestive, and autoimmune conditions, such as:
- Alzheimer's disease
- Anxiety and depression
- Asthma
- Cancer
- Dementia
- Dysmenorrhea and PMS
- Herpes
- High blood pressure and elevated cholesterol
- Parkinson's disease
- Acne
- Chronic fatigue
- Chronic constipation
- Irritable bowel syndrome
- Obesity

Coaching Tip

Ayurveda is an approach that focuses on the application of different mind-body techniques in order to heal the body. The healing process will vary depending upon the distinctive characteristics and needs of each client. If one of your clients is interested in getting an Ayurvedic approach coaching, you might want to refer him or her to an Ayurvedic lifestyle certified practitioner. Furthermore, if your client wants to enrich a self-care lifestyle by practicing one of the complementary Ayurvedic approaches (like massage therapy or acupuncture), it would be helpful for you to have a directory resource with a list of skillful practitioners around the area. You can always expand your education, and might find yourself naturally interested in learning more about Ayurveda by getting a complimentary certification.

Contraindications

- Pregnancy
- Fever
- Acute illness
- Open sores
- Dehydration
- Intoxication

It is important to make sure you are not recommending that your clients replace conventional care with Ayurveda. They should not stop visiting their healthcare providers when they start following any Ayurveda approach. Your provider will want to be aware of any possible side effects that occur when following any Ayurvedic approach (including diet, cleansing techniques and massage). Some Ayurvedic products or herbs could potentially be toxic. Many Ayurvedic products are regulated as dietary supplements instead of conventional medicines because they have not been required to meet the same standards for safety.

Research and Benefits

Most Ayurvedic studies have been small in size and have not been well designed or have lacked control groups, which affects research results. While the scientific research methodologies have not been robust, there is a long history of traditional safe and effective usage, and that body of historical evidence continues to support one of the oldest systems of healing in the world.

Most of the current studies are reductionistic, investigating the effectiveness of a specific Ayurvedic herbal compound, and they fail to account for the overall synergistic impact of how an Ayurvedic practitioner actually works with dietary changes, movement, massage, cleansing treatments, herbs, and meditation. Nonetheless, a clinical trial funded by the National Center for Complementary and Integrative Health (NCCIH) found that Ayurvedic herbal compounds had comparable effectiveness to conventional allopathic pharmaceutical treatments for osteoarthritis (Vishal). One of the most studied Ayurvedic herbs is turmeric, which has proven to be significantly effective with inflammatory conditions, such as arthritis, and with some digestive disorders. Frankincense has similarly been shown to have anti-inflammatory effects and help lower pain levels when it is consumed.

Practitioner Training and Credentials

There are a few approved Ayurvedic schools in the US; however, there is no license offered for Ayurvedic practitioners. Instead, many Ayurvedic practitioners get licensed in complementary health care fields such as massage or midwifery. More information regarding the credentials, training, regulation, and licensing of complementary health practitioners can be found at the NCCIH website.

Resources

You can find more information about how to practice an Ayurvedic lifestyle and how you can become an Ayurveda practitioner at the Chopra Center website, the National Center for Biotechnology Information, the California College of Ayurveda, and the Ayurvedic Institute.

References

Axe, J. "Seven benefits of Ayurvedic Medicine." In *Food is Medicine.* N.p., 2016. draxe.com/food-is-medicine. Accessed April 2017

Chopra, D. "What Is Ayurveda?" The Chopra Center. N.p., 2016. chopra.com/articles/what-is-ayurveda. Accessed April 2017.

Guha, Á. "What Happens on a Visit to an Ayurvedic Practitioner?" *Taking Charge of Your Health and Wellbeing.* University of Minnesota, 2016.

Ayurvedic Medicine: In Depth. National Center for Complementary and Integrative Health. N.p., 2017. nccih.nih.gov/health/ayurveda/introduction.htm. Accessed April 2017.

Ayurvedic Medicine: In Depth. National Center for Complementary and Integrative Health. N.p., 2017. nccih.nih.gov/health/ayurveda/introduction.htm. Accessed April 2017

Patwardhan, B, Vaidya, A, & Chorghde, M. "Ayurveda and Natural Products Drug Discovery." (n.d.). researchgate.net/publication/228421013_Ayurveda_and_natural_produ cts_discovery. Accessed April 2017.

Vishal, AA, Mishra, A, & Raychaudhuri, SP. A double blind, randomized, placebo controlled clinical study evaluates the early efficacy of aflapin in subjects with osteoarthritis of knee. International Journal of Medical Sciences. 2011;8(7):615-622.

BREATHWORK—DIAPHRAGMATIC BREATHING
Elaine Santos

Diaphragmatic breathing is the most basic relaxation technique. It involves breathing from the lower stomach or abdomen rather than from the thoracic or chest area. Diaphragmatic breathing is often paired with other relaxation techniques like autogenic training, progressive muscular relaxation, and mental imagery. Breathing is an involuntary process that can be controlled. Diaphragmatic breathing is a simple and powerful tool for stress relief.

History
Breathing as a therapeutic practice can be traced back thousands of years to the ancient practices of yoga and Tai'Chi Chuan; diaphragmatic breathing is an integral component to both disciplines. In yoga, the breathing element is called pranayama, a Sanskrit term that translates to restoring one's vital life force of energy (Seaward, 369). The connection between the therapeutic power of breathing and higher consciousness has also been explored since ancient times through meditation.

In the 1960s, breathwork therapy developed with the focus on expanding consciousness and releasing trauma. The main schools of breathwork include Holotropic Breathwork, Rebirthing, and Clarity Breathwork (which evolved from Rebirthing). Practitioners are certified and facilitate one-on-one or group sessions and use circular breathing. The philosophy is that breathwork can help release blocked energy and support healing (goodtherapy.org).

Philosophy
Stress affects breathing. When a stressful occurrence happens, the body's sympathetic nervous system, often referred to as the fight or flight response, activates. The sympathetic nervous system is one half of the autonomic nervous system; the parasympathetic is the other half. The autonomic nervous system controls the body's involuntary functions such as breathing, heartbeat, and digestion. A number of physiological reactions take place during a stress response including: blood pressure and heart rate increase, digestion halts, blood is rushed to the extremities, eyes dilate, and breathing becomes shallow and contained in the chest. Some people hold their breath in a stress state and that also triggers those same physiological responses.

Diaphragmatic breathing activates the parasympathetic nervous system, which opposes the sympathetic nervous system. When one is activated the other is quiet. Through longer exhalations, the relaxation response is triggered; heart rate and blood pressure decrease, digestion processes resume, pupils contract, pressure is off the thoracic cavity, and the sympathetic drive decreases. Breathing becomes deeper and tension is released through diaphragmatic breathing.

Another explanation of how diaphragmatic breathing works to create relaxation is related to vibrations of the heart. Itzhak Bentov's (1988) theory is that the force of contractions of the left ventricle and the blood sends a vibration through the aorta that reverberates through the body. A pause in the breathing cycle stops this reverberation. Diaphragmatic breathing accents long pauses decreasing the resonance, which creates a calming effect (Seaward).

Treatments: What to Expect

Diaphragmatic breathing is simple and can be broken down into three steps. First, get into a comfortable position, sitting or lying down. Next is concentration. Minimize external interruptions by closing out as much noise as possible. The second part of concentration is minimizing internal interruptions. Focus attention on breathing and letting go of distracting thoughts. Common strategies include letting go of thoughts when exhaling, focus on each phase of the breath (inhale, pause, exhale, pause), and focusing specifically on the exhale. It is recommended to inhale and exhale through the nose, if possible. Visualization, the last step, is optional. It is often helpful to include visualization in breathing to help with concentration. One common visual is to imagine breathing in fresh air and exhaling a cloud. First the cloud will be dark, but as the breathing continues, the cloud becomes clearer and clearer. (Seaward)

Setting: anywhere (in the car, dental chair, office desk, etc.), or in facilitator's studio/office.

Duration: ~1 hour.

Cost: Free. Professional sessions, up to $200.

Best Suited for These Conditions

- Muscle tension
- Stress
- Back pain
- Migraine
- Anxiety

Coaching Tip

Consider being trained in professional breathwork sessions for additional skill and knowledge about its benefits and values. But even without that extra training, as a coach, you can always introduce a few moments of centered, calming breathwork at the onset or during a coaching session to help the client feel grounded, present, and emotionally calm. Ask the client to place one hand on the chest over the heart and one on the belly, and simply notice the inhalations and exhalations for a minute or two. Guide the client to gently move the breath from the diaphragm.

Contraindications

- If a client has emphysema (chronic obstructive pulmonary disease—COPD) or asthma, have them consult with their doctor
- Hyperventilation
- Dizziness

Research and Benefits

- Decreases resting heart rate
- Promotes feelings of relaxation
- Decreases muscle tension
- Improves mental clarity
- Increases oxygen capacity in lungs
- Helps deal with stress overload
- Chronic pain/lower back pain

Diaphragmatic breathing research shows success in reducing pain including childbirth (Lamaze), chronic lower back pain, and migraine. Other studies show digestion improvement and stress reduction. Research is inconclusive on whether diaphragmatic breathing is beneficial to those with asthma or COPD.

Practitioner Training and Credentials

An individual can practice this technique on their own. If clients want to learn more breathing techniques, they can attend yoga classes. If clients are interested in breathwork therapy, they should work with a certified breathwork practitioner.

Resources

Eric Franklin's free video on breathing—franklinmethod.com/latest-news/enjoy-your-breath-enjoy-your-life

Yoga Journal is a good resource on pranayama:—yogajournal.com/article/practice-section/healing-breath

This website has articles on different therapies including breathwork—goodtherapy.org/learn-about-therapy/types/breathwork

Clarity and Holotropic Breathwork—claritybreathwork.com/overview-of-clarity-breathwork

holotropic.com/about.shtml

References

Claritybreathwork.com. claritybreathwork.com/overview-of-clarity-breathwork/. Accessed 9 April 2017.

Ernst, E. "Breathing techniques—adjunctive treatment modalities for asthma? A systematic review." *European Respiratory Journal* 15 (2000) 969–972.

Franklin, E. *Dynamic Alignment Through Imagery*, 2nd ed. Champaign, IL: Human Kinetics, 2012.

Franklin, E. *Relax your Neck Liberate your Shoulders*. Elysian Editions, 2002.

Goodtherapy.com. 9 May 2016, goodtherapy.org/learn-about-therapy/types/breathwork. Accessed 10 April 2017.

Kaushik, R, Kaushik, RM, Mahajan, SK, & Rajesh, V. (2005). "Biofeedback assisted diaphragmatic breathing and systematic relaxation versus propranolol in long term prophylaxis of migraine." *Complementary Therapies in Medicine* 13, no. 3 (2005): 165–174.

Jerath, R, Edry, J, Barnes, VA, & Jerath, V. "Physiology of long pranayamic breathing: Neural respiratory elements may provide a mechanism that explains how slow deep breathing shifts the autonomic nervous system." *Med. Hypotheses*, 67, no. 3 (Apr 18, 2006): 566-71. Epub.

Sapolsky, RM. *Why Zebras Don't Get Ulcers.* 3rd ed. St. Martin's Griffin, 2004.

Seaward, B. *Managing Stress*. 8th Edition. Jones and Bartlett, 2015.

Todd, M. *The Thinking Body: A Study of the Balancing Forces of Dynamic Man*, The Gestalt Journal Press, 1937.

Vitacca, M, Cini, E, Bianchi, L, & Ambrosino, N. "Acute Effects of Deep Diaphragmatic Breathing in COPD Patients with Chronic Respiratory Insufficiency." *European Respiratory Journal* 11,1998, 408–415.

CHIROPRACTIC

Michael Craigen

Chiropractic is a system of medicine that focuses on diagnosis of joint and spinal column misalignments, and manipulative treatment to restore balance and support healing of the entire body. Chiropractic posits that alignment of bodily structures has significant and numerous effects on the health of organs, nerves, muscles, tendons and ligaments.

History

The word "chiropractic" stems from its Greek words "cheir" and "praktos," which means "treatment done by hand" (Dagenais & Haldeman). Daniel David Palmer, known as "the father of chiropractic," began the practice in 1895, performing the first documented chiropractic adjustment in Davenport, Iowa (Keating). Palmer claimed the recipient, who had recently lost his hearing after hearing his back "pop," regained his hearing the day after the adjustment (Palmer). Palmer went on to found the first school dedicated to teaching these concepts in 1897, known as the Palmer School of Chiropractic (Palmer). Chiropractic continued to expand across the country and into other parts of the world, with new schools forming throughout the 20th century (Keating). Early chiropractors faced backlash from the medical community after the 1910 Flexner Report declared competing systems of medicine (naturopaths, chiropractors, and homeopaths) to be nonscientific and illegitimate. Over the next century, the chiropractic field closed gaps in its knowledge base, strengthened its education and training, and regained credibility due to comparative effectiveness trials that focused on what chiropractic does best. Today just under fifteen percent of the public reports having received chiropractic care. In recent years, an extensive body of research on the practice and theories surrounding chiropractic has developed, and it is now one of the largest alternative medicine practices in the Western world (Kaptchuk & Eisenberg), with over 60,000 practicing in the US in a multi-billion dollar industry (Ernst).

Philosophy

Chiropractic is primarily concerned with the alignment of the spine and its impact on overall functioning of the body because the spine is a central part of the musculoskeletal and nervous systems (Horowitz). The foundations of chiropractic can be dated back to antiquity in practices such as bone setting, mentioned in ancient medical texts (Horowtiz), which influenced early chiropractors in the 19th century (Kaptchuk and Eisenberg). Palmer's early fundamental dogma emphasized that all disease can be traced back to vertebral subluxation, or misalignment of the spine (Palmer). Then, through correcting misalignments and allowing nerves to operate freely without obstruction, the innate intelligence of body would heal itself (Keating).

Practitioners who strictly believed like Palmer that this was the root of all illness were known as "straights," while the "mixers" branched off and began integrating elements of other forms of medicine. Modern day philosophy embraces a more holistic viewpoint (Mootz) that factors in scientific findings (Keating), combined with some elements of tradition (Smith). Many chiropractors now take on a variety of approaches in the healing process, often overlapping with other forms of treatment such as physical therapy, utilizing many techniques from massage, myofascial release, and homeopathy (Kaptchuk & Eisenberg).

Treatments: What to Expect

- Spinal manipulation therapy (chiropractic adjustment)
- Consultation
- Anatomical mechanics
- Physical strength/fitness
- Nutrition/Lifestyle
- Corrective exercise training
- Trigger point therapy/myofascial release
- Ultrasound, laser, and other electrophysical agents

Setting: Chiropractor's office with specialized equipment.
Duration: 15–60 minutes
Cost: $65–150

Best Suited for These Conditions

- Spinal pain/discomfort
- Sciatica
- Fibromyalgia
- Chronic pain
- Muscle tension and spasms
- Headaches

Coaching Tip

Given the wide variety of techniques and approaches in chiropractic today, coaches are advised to invite clients to do their research on local chiropractors and familiarize themselves with their backgrounds and styles. Since poor biomechanics are often the cause of cumulative spinal injuries, clients should also be directed towards chiropractors or other professionals who can emphasize biomechanical correction and muscular stability when necessary. Leaders in the field urge chiropractic be considered as a low cost, non-pharmacological treatment to reduce back pain, especially in the face of the opioid crisis.

Contraindications

- Osteoporosis
- Fractures, dislocations
- Vertebral artery stenosis
- Some arthritic conditions (such as rheumatoid arthritis)
- Various malignancies/tumors
- Localized conditions that may be affected by manipulation

Research

The US National Center for Complementary and Integrative Health (NCCIH) supported research on chiropractic care that found patient satisfaction was high compared to conventional medical care for management of low back pain. The Center also supports further research at the Palmer Center for Chiropractic Research. In 2018, the largest randomized clinical trial (RCT) in chiropractic concluded that chiropractic care resulted in better short-term improvements in low back pain intensity and pain-related disability than conventional medical care (Goertz). Prior to this clinical trial, independent chiropractic research findings were criticized in one review (Ernst), but that review also underwent criticism (Morley), threatening validity of its conclusions (Bronfort). A long history of debates and back-and-forth turf battles should give you some idea of the continuous struggle that chiropractors engage in, as they attempt to establish a foothold as trusted partners in integrative medicine.

Low Back Pain: There is strong evidence that spinal manipulation aids in chronic low back pain in adults, and moderate evidence in its ability to treat acute back pain (Bronfort; Chou; Goertz). A systematic review in 2010 showed significant effects in pain and mobility that either equaled or surpassed other treatments (Dagenais). A 2013 randomized control trial found that 12 spinal manipulation sessions amounted to the ideal amount of treatments (Haas). In a 2014 randomized controlled trial comparing chiropractic and standard medical care, chiropractic was more effective at reducing short-term pain (Schneider). As stated above, in 2018 the largest RCT in chiropractic history provided groundbreaking results on comparative effectiveness of chiropractic over conventional medical care for low back pain reduction among US service members (Goertz).

Sciatica/Radiculopathy: A systematic review and meta-analysis in 2013 showed significantly higher rates of healing sciatica in comparison to standard treatments (Lewis). Other systematic reviews suggested possible effectiveness in treating lumbar radiculopathy and disk herniation-related radiculopathy (Leninger).

Neck Pain: A 2008 best evidence synthesis found spinal manipulation in combination with exercise was more effective in treating than non-invasive treatments (Hurwitz). A 2012 randomized control trial found spinal manipulation was more efficacious in both the long and short-term at treating acute and sub-acute neck pain (Bronfort). A 2004 meta-analysis found the spinal manipulations could be effective in improving mobility in mechanical neck issues (Gross). A 2004 systematic review showed moderate evidence of spinal manipulation and mobilization's ability to reduce short-term pain in chronic cases of neck pain (Bronfort).

Asthma, Allergy, and other conditions: A 2007 systematic review showed some evidence in asthma, cervicogenic vertigo, and infantile colic benefitting from chiropractic care, as well as children with otitis media and elderly with pneumonia (Hawk). A 2010 systematic review showed statistically insignificant results in treating asthma, recommending it be used as a supplementary therapy (Kaminskyi). One pilot study found that realignment of the C1/atlas vertebra is associated with sustained blood pressure reduction similar to two drug therapy (Bakris).

Fibromyalgia: A 2009 systematic review by Ernst shows no evidence that spinal adjustments aid in treating fibromyalgia (Ernst). A 2015 systematic overview of reviews showed a need for more research on CAM practices and their effectiveness in treating fibromyalgia, specifying chiropractic and other treatment philosophies as having inconsistent results (Lauche). In a 2009 randomized control trial on women with fibromyalgia, chiropractic treatment increased adherence to exercise regimen that improved individuals' states (Paton).

Tension-type Headaches: There is some evidence that spinal manipulation can aid in relieving headaches (Bryans; Bronfort). A 2011 systematic review showed spinal manipulation was as efficacious as drugs like propranolol in treating tension-type headaches (Chalibi). A 2017 critical review claimed insufficiency in the research of manual therapy and headaches, highlighting the need for investment in reliable testing (Moore). Similarly, a 2006 review showed no evidence that manual therapies have a positive influence on tension-type headache (Fernandez).

Practitioner Training and Credentials
The World Health Organization's mandate for chiropractor training dictates that those without prior healthcare education or experience must complete 4200 hours of student/teacher contact in a 4-year degree program, with at least 1000 of those dedicated to supervised clinical training.

The educational models throughout the world vary, but most paths involve the either completion of a bachelor's degree in a scientific subject that leads into chiropractic school, a 5-year degree-program that trains one as a chiropractor, or a chiropractic/health-science degree followed by a pre-professional master's level program. Healthcare professionals with prior experience can accelerate chiropractic training depending on their previous work and education, or can obtain limited chiropractic educational qualification through satisfying the minimum requirements on a part-time basis.

Other programs may train an individual for limited qualification to perform basic chiropractic techniques safely. In the US, boards of chiropractic examiners operate with state governments, issuing the official license to practice to qualified applicants who graduate from accredited programs and successfully pass the national board examinations, administered by the National Board of Chiropractic Examiners.

Resources
American Chiropractic Association—acatoday.org.
Spine-health—spine-health.com.
World Health Organization's "Basic Training for Chiropractic" manual—
    apps.who.int/medicinedocs/en/m/abstract/Js14076e.

References
Bakris, G, et al. "Atlas vertebra realignment and achievement of arterial pressure goal in hypertensive patients: a pilot study." *Journal of Human Hypertension,* 21, no. 5 (2007): 347-52, doi: 10.1038/sj.jhh.1002133.

Bronfort, G, et al. "Non-invasive physical treatments for chronic/recurrent headache." *Cochrane Database of Systematic Reviews,* 3 (2004): doi: 10.1002/14651858.CD001878.pub2

Bronfort, G, et al. "Efficacy of spinal manipulation and mobilization for low back pain and neck pain: a systematic review and best evidence synthesis." *Spine Journal,* 4, no. 3, (2004): 335-356, doi: 10.1016/j.spinee.2003.06.002

Bronfort, G, et al. "Effectiveness of manual therapies: the UK evidence report." *Chiropractic & Manual Therapies,* 18, no. 1 (2010): 3.

Bronfort, G, et al. "Spinal Manipulation, Medication, or Home Exercise with Advice for Acute and Subacute Neck PainA Randomized Trial." *Annals of Internal Medicine,* 156, no. 1 Part 1 (2012): 1-10.

Bryans, R, et al. "Evidence-based guidelines for the chiropractic treatment of adults with headache." *Journal of manipulative and physiological therapeutics* 34 no. 5 (2011): 274-289.

Canter, PH & Ernst, E. "Sources of bias in reviews of spinal manipulation for back pain." *Weiner Klinische Wochenschrift,* 117 (2005): 333-41.

Chalibi, A, et al. "Manual therapies for migraine: a systematic review." *Journal of Headache and Pain,* 12, no. 2 (2011): 127-33, doi: 10.1007/s10194-011-0296-6

Chapman-Smith, DA, Cleveland, CS III. "International status, standards, and education of the chiropractic profession." *Principles and Practice of Chiropractic,* 3rd ed., Scott Haldeman et al. McGraw-Hill, 2005.

Chou, R & Huffman, LH. "Nonpharmacologic therapies for acute and chronic low back pain: a review of the evidence for an American Pain Society/American College of Physicians clinical practice guideline." *Annals of Internal Medicine,* 147, no. 7 (2007): 492-504.

Dagenais, S & Haldeman, S. "Chiropractic." *Primary Care: Clinics in Office Practice,* 29, no. 2 (2002): 419-437, doi: 10.1016/S0095-4543(01)00005-7

Dagenais, S, Gay, RE, Tricco, AC, Freeman, MD, & Mayer, JM. "NASS contemporary concepts in spine care: spinal manipulation therapy for acute low back pain." *The Spine Journal,* 10, no. 10 (2010): 918-40. doi: 10.1016/j.spinee.2010.07.389

Ernst, E. "Chiropractic: a critical evaluation." *Journal of Pain and Symptom Management,* 35, no. 5 (2008): 544-62.

Ernst, E. "Chiropractic treatment for fibromyalgia: a systematic review." *Clinical Rheumatology,*28, no. 10 (2009): 1175-1178.

Ernst, E. "Deaths after chiropractic: a review of published cases." *International Journal of Clinical Practice,* 64, no. 8 (2010): 1162-1165, doi: 10.1111/j.1742-1241.2010.02352.x

Fernández-de-Las-Peñas, C, et al. "Are manual therapies effective in reducing pain from tension-type headache? A systematic review." *Clinical Journal of Pain,* 22, no. 3,:((2006): 278-85 doi: 10.1097/01.ajp.0000173017.64741.86.

Goertz, C, et al. "Effect of Usual Medical Care Plus Chiropractic Care vs Usual Medial Care Alone on Pain and Disability Among US Service Members with Low Back Pain: A Comparative effectiveness clinical trial. *JAMA Network Open.* (2018): 1(1);e180105.309:10.1001/jamanetworkopen.2018.0105

Gross, A, et al. "Manipulation or mobilisation for neck pain: a Cochrane review." *Musculoskeletal Science & Practice,* 15, no. 4 (2010): 315-33, doi: 10.1016/j.math.2010.04.002

Haas, M, et al. "Dose-response and efficacy of spinal manipulation for care of chronic low back pain: a randomized controlled trial." *The Spine Journal* 14 no. 7 (2014): 1106-1116.

Hawk, C, et al. "Chiropractic care for nonmusculoskeletal conditions: a systematic review with implications for whole systems research."

Journal of Alternative and Complementary Medicine, 13, no. 5 (2007): 491-512, doi: 10.1089/acm.2007.7088

Horowitz, S. "Evidence-based applications for chiropractic." *Alternative and Complementary Therapies,* 13, no. 5 (2007): 248-253. doi: 10.1089/act.2007.13505.

Hurwitz, EL, et al. "Treatment of neck pain: noninvasive interventions: results of the Bone and Joint Decade 2000–2010 Task Force on Neck Pain and Its Associated Disorders." *Journal of manipulative and physiological therapeutics* 32.2 (2009): S141-S175.

Kaminskyj, A, et al. "Chiropractic care for patients with asthma: a systematic review of the literature." *Journal of the Canadian Chiropractic Association,* 54, no. 1 (2010): 24-32, PMCID: PMC2829683.

Kaptchuk, TJ & Eisenberg, DM. "Chiropractic: origins, controversies, and contributions." *Archives of Internal Medicine,* 158, no. 20, (1998): 2215-2224. doi: 10.1001/archinte.158.20.2215

Keating, JC, Cleveland, CS, & Menke, MJ. "Chiropractic history: a primer." *Association for the History of Chiropractic,* 2004.

Keating, JC. "A brief history of the chiropractic profession." *Principles and Practices of Chiropractic,* by Scott Haldeman, McGraw-Hill: 2005, 23-63.

Keating, JC. "Philosophy in chiropractic." *Principles and Practices of Chiropractic,* by Scott Haldeman, McGraw-Hill, 2005, 77-98.

Lauche, R, et al. "A systematic overview of reviews for complementary and alternative therapies in the treatment of the fibromyalgia syndrome." *Evidence-Based Complementary and Alternative Medicine,* 2015 (2015): doi: 10.1155/2015/610615

Lewis, RA, et al. "Comparative clinical effectiveness of management strategies for sciatica: a systematic review and network meta-analyses." *Spine Journal,* 15, no. 6 (2013): 1461-77, doi: 10.1016/j.spinee.2013.08.049.

Leninger, B, et al. "Spinal manipulation or mobilization fro radiculopathy: a systematic review." *Physical Medicine and Rehabilitation Clinics of North America,* 22, no. 1 (2010): 105-125, doi: 10.1016/j.pmr.2010.11.002.

McGill, SM, et al. "Coordination of muscle activity to assure stability of the lumbar spine." *Journal of electromyography and kinesiology* 13.4 (2003): 353-359.

Mootz, RD & Phillips, RB. Chiropractic belief systems. *Chiropractic in the United States: Training Practice, and Research,* by Daniel C. Cherkin and Robert D. Mootz, Agency for Health Care Policy and Research, (1997): 9-16.

Morley, J; Rosner, AL, & Redwood, L. "A case study of misrepresentation of the scientific literature: recent reviews of chiropractic." *Journal of Alternative and Complementary Medicine,* 7, no. 1 (2004): 65-78, doi: 10.1089/107555301300004547.

Palmer, DD. *The Science, Art and Philosophy of Chiropractic.* Portland Printing House Company, 1910.

Paton, LB, et al. "Effects of resistance training and chiropractic treatment in women with fibromyalgia." *Journal of Alternative and Complementary Medicine,* 15, no. 3 (2009): 21-8, doi: 10.1089/acm.2008.0132.

Posadzki, P & Ernst, E. "Spinal manipulation: an update of a systematic review of systemic reviews." *New Zealand Medical Journal,* 124, no. 1340 (2011): 55-71. PMID: 21952385.

Smith, M & Carber, LA. "Survey of US chiropractor attitudes and behaviors about subluxation." *Journal of Chiropractic Humanities,* 15 (2008): 19-26. doi: 10.1016/S1556-3499(13)60166-7.

Schneider, M, et al. "A comparison of chiropractic manipulation methods and usual medical care for low back pain: a randomized control clinical trial." *Journal of Alternative and Complementary Medicine,* 20, no. 5 (2014): A22-3.

World Health Organization "Basic training and safety in chiropractic." *World Health Organization,* 2005, apps.who.int/medicinedocs/en/m/abstract/Js14076e. Accessed May 2017.

CRANIOSACRAL THERAPY
Emilie Miller

Craniosacral therapy involves gentle manipulation of the cranial bones while sensing and directing the cerebrospinal pulse that is detected at the base of the sacrum and the occiput or back of the head.

History

Craniosacral therapy has its roots in the medical field of osteopathy. Osteopathy is the treatment of medical conditions via manipulation and realignment of the muscle tissue and bones of the body, so as to restore sound biomechanics. The development of osteopathy is credited to Andrew Taylor Still. In Missouri, in 1892, Still opened the American School of Osteopathy. Craniosacral therapy links back to cranial osteopathy, as discovered in the 1930s and named by Dr. William Sutherland, a graduate of the American School of Osteopathy. Sutherland, like all physicians during his time, had been taught to believe that the eight bones in the cranium were fused together and immovable. However, while a student, and then in the time that followed, Sutherland observed that the cranial bones did in fact allow for movement. In further experimentation, Sutherland confirmed movement in the bones of the cranium and also observed that their movement was linked to movement and adjustment in the sacrum. By the 1940s, Sutherland had created a course called Osteopathy in the Cranial Field at the American School of Osteopathy.

John Upledger, a doctor of osteopathy, was the person responsible for developing and then naming the therapeutic modality craniosacral therapy. Upledger did so in the 1970s. He was introduced to the idea of motion in the cranial bones by one of Sutherland's protégés, Harold Magoun, DO, at the Osteopathic Cranial Academy, as established by Sutherland in 1947. This was the beginning of a period when Upledger studied under Magoun.

While a research fellow at the Faculty of Osteopathic Medicine at Michigan State University, Upledger and colleagues conducted clinical experiments that proved Sutherland's findings of cranial bone movement, as well as the cranium's connection to the sacrum via membranes and cerebrospinal fluid (CSF). The craniosacral matrix of protective membranes and cerebrospinal fluid is what Upledger called the craniosacral system. The craniosacral system extends from the bones of the face and skull, down into the sacrum and tailbone.

Upledger eventually left Michigan State University in order to found the Upledger Institute. The Upledger Institute trains non-doctors of osteopathy, and since the trainees are not doctors, Upledger adjusted the name from cranial osteopathy to craniosacral therapy.

Philosophy

According to craniosacral therapy, and cranial osteopathy, the significance of the cranial bones' movement and their ability to be minutely adjusted is that the ability to properly align the bones around the brain, which are also in close proximity to the spinal cord, to facilitate improved functioning of the central nervous system. Craniosacral therapy purports that when the central nervous system is alleviated from stress, natural healing throughout the body can occur. Shifts in the cranial bones, by a craniosacral therapist, can release any impingements in the flow or rhythm of the cerebrospinal fluid. When the protective cerebrospinal fluid is flowing unrestricted, nerve conductivity is enhanced and natural, restorative responses are elicited by the body's systems, including the central nervous system. Communication among the body's systems is unobstructed and, with less effort, the body is able to return to homeostasis after encountering disruptive external stimuli.

Treatments: What to Expect

A craniosacral therapy session should be administered by a therapist who is certified in craniosacral therapy. There are resources at the end of this section that will assist clients in locating a certified craniosacral therapist.

It is advisable to seek out a therapist who has been in practice for at least a few years. Should a client be scheduling a craniosacral session for a specific reason, i.e., low back pain, migraines, etc., it would be helpful to locate a craniosacral therapist who has a background in specifically treating the client's condition. During the session, the therapist will be using his or her hands to lightly touch the client's body, most often at, but not limited to, the head and sacrum region. The therapist will be using their hands to get a sense of the rhythms of the body, as well as where the body holds tension, or is even trapped in tension. Depending on the needs of the client's body, the therapist will use gentle pressure with their hands to initiate soft tissue release, structural decompression and mobilization, lymphatic flow, and somatoemotional release (Kailas).

Setting: Private office, table similar to massage therapist's.
Duration: 60–90 minutes.
Cost: $80–$140, typically not covered by health insurance.

Best Suited for These Conditions

- Scoliosis
- Chronic pain
- Depression

- Allergies
- Chronic neck and back pain
- Migraines
- Motor-coordination impairments
- Learning disabilities
- PTSD
- Anxiety and stress
- Spinal cord injuries
- Headaches
- PTSD
- Connective tissue disorders
- TMJ
- Chronic traumatic encephalopathy

This list is not all-inclusive of the conditions craniosacral therapy is said to treat and/or alleviate. To find a more exhaustive list, please visit the Upledger Institute's website: Upledger.com

Coaching Tip

Advise the client, when looking for craniosacral therapists, it is important to note where they were certified (if the certifying organization is not recognized, be sure to research its legitimacy), if their certification is current, what other certifications they might have, and if they are familiar with the conditions the client is hoping to treat via craniosacral therapy. Most importantly, do they and their place of practice exude comfort and safety.

Contraindications

- Traumatic brain injury
- Stroke
- Brain hemorrhage
- Tumor
- Rheumatoid arthritis
- Recent spinal tap
- Down syndrome
- Arnold-Chiari Malformation (defects in the cerebellum)

Research and Benefits

Research on the effectiveness of craniosacral therapy was conducted at Oxford Brookes University in the UK in 2012. This particular study generated "positive clinical outcomes" in which "pain reduction and improvement in general wellbeing of patients" (Jäkel & von Hauenschild). However, the study concluded that more research on craniosacral therapy was necessary before it could be recommended for clinical use.

The practice of craniosacral therapy is one of controversy among health and therapeutic practitioners. It has been dismissed as "pseudoscience" (Atwood). The speculation about craniosacral therapy's legitimacy is mostly because of the lack of research on the therapy and due to the subtle effects of craniosacral therapy being too difficult to measure. However, as adduced among the list of articles and studies on the Upledger Institute's website, research on craniosacral therapy is ongoing. The research studies published on their website unequivocally conclude that craniosacral therapy is a viable, effective, therapeutic modality.

The Upledger Institute cites one 2016 study conducted by regenerative medicine clinic, Regenexx (Regenexx.com). The participants in the study were chosen due to their indication of neck pain. As part of the study, all of the participants were blindfolded and told that they would be receiving craniosacral therapy to treat their neck pain. However, half of the participants received craniosacral therapy and the other half received a sham treatment (Centeno). The results showed that not only did those receiving authentic craniosacral therapy report a reduction in their pain, they also had increased mobility in their neck. The control group saw less to little improvement.

The Upledger Institute's website provides an additional thirty-three studies supporting the efficacy of craniosacral therapy. The studies provided not only draw favorable conclusions about craniosacral therapy's ability to provide relief, but many of them also highlight the non-invasive nature of craniosacral therapy. For many, the lack of injections, elimination of exposure to radiation, and reduced use of pharmaceuticals, makes craniosacral therapy an appealing therapeutic alternative.

Practitioner Training and Credentials

The Upledger Institute offers a Craniosacral Therapy Certification Program. The program is open to those who are already licensed in a hands-on therapeutic technique, as the Institute's program does not offer that type of licensure. There are two levels of craniosacral therapy certification offered, the second level being more advanced. A practitioner may take just the first level, or both. Within each level are three examination phases. The successful passing of the first level, or both levels, awards the participant with their craniosacral certification. Once certified, therapists must maintain their certification by completing 24 hours of Upledger Institute-approved continuing education every four years.

Certification applications can be found on the Institute's website, along with continuing education options—upledger.com/therapies/certification-programs.php

The Biodynamic Craniosacral Therapy Association of North America (BCTA/NA) also offers a certification program in which those who complete the program successfully, graduate as Registered Craniosacral Therapists (RCST®). Based in Youngsville, NC, the BCTA/NA's program is a 700-hour certification, which includes 350 classroom hours, practicum, sessions provided by an RCST, a research paper or presentation, and independent study. Each training includes no more than 6 participants. Once having completed and graduated from the BCTA/NA's training program, the association has in place guidelines for RCST to remain approved and in good standing. Information on training to become a Registered Craniosacral Therapist through the Biodynamic Craniosacral Therapy Association can be found at craniosacraltherapy.org/teacher-approval-criteria

Resources

The Biodynamic Craniosacral Therapy Association of North America—
    craniosacraltherapy.org
The Upledger Institute—upledger.com
Both organizations offer information on craniosacral therapy, assistance in
    locating a craniosacral therapist, and information on craniosacral
    training for professionals.
The Osteopathic Cranial Academy—cranialacademy.org
Kate MacKinnon—kmackinnon.com
Wellness Institute—wellnessinstitute.net

References

Atwood, KC. "Naturopathy, Pseudoscience, and Medicine: Myths and
    Fallacies vs Truth." *Medscape General Medicine Journal* 6, no. 1
    (2004). ncbi.nlm.nih.gov/pmc/articles/PMC1140750. Accessed March
    and April 2017.
*The Biodynamic Craniosacral Association of North America Family of
    Sites*. craniosacraltherapy.org. Accessed March and April 2017.
Centeno, C. "New Craniosacral Therapy Research—This Duck Doesn't
    Quack Anymore." *Regenexx* August 30, 2016.
    iahe.com/images/pdf/NEW_CranioSacral_Research.pdf. Accessed
    March & April, 2017.
Craniosacral Research Blog. Biodynamic Health Systems.
    biodynamichealth.com/craniosacral-research. Accessed March and
    April 2017.
Irish Association of Craniosacral Therapists Family of Sites.
    iacst.ie/index.php. Accessed March and April 2017.

Jakel, A & von Hauenschild, P. "A Systematic Review to Evaluate the Clinical Benefits of Craniosacral Therapy." *Complementary Therapies in Medicine* 20, no. 6 (2012). doi: 10.1016/j.ctim.2012.07.009. Accessed March and April 2017.

Kailas. "The Clinical Applications of CranioSacral Therapy." *Craniosacral Topics*, January 8, 2009. craniosacraltopics.blogspot.com/2009/01/clinical-applications-of-craniosacral.html. Accessed March and April 2017.

MacKinnon, K. *From My Hands and Heart.* Hay House, 2014.

The Upledger Institute Family of Sites. The Upledger Institute International. upledger.com/index.php. Accessed March and April 2017.

Upledger, JE. *Craniosacral Therapy: What It Is, How It Works.* North Atlantic Books, 2008.

CURANDERISMO
Meckell Milburn

Curanderismo is a traditional Mesoamerican system of healing that consists of various modalities used to treat mental, physical, spiritual, and emotional maladies. Healers in this tradition are called curanderas or curanderos. They use techniques that include prayer, herbs, energy cleansing, massage, and heart-to-heart talks in their healing practice.

History

Curanderismo was created and is practiced in what is present-day Mexico and Central America, and the southwestern United States. The indigenous cultures from this area, including the Aztecan, Mayan, and Incan cultures, believed in maintaining harmony with nature and its importance to body, soul, spirit, and emotions. Montezuma I, an Aztecan emperor in the 1500s, developed the Huaxtepec Garden with thousands of medicinal plants used for study and research that led to knowledge of and expertise with herbal remedies. Although the Spanish conquistadors, claiming blasphemy, destroyed much of this research, vast amounts of knowledge of herbs and other natural medicinal resources were still passed down from generation to generation.

With the arrival of Spanish missionaries in the 1600s, the Catholic religion was introduced. Catholicism played an important role in Curanderismo, by contributing the prayers to Catholic saints and the religious artifacts that are now widely used throughout Curanderismo. Around this time, European ideologies around witchcraft, superstition, and supernatural influences began framing the belief that many ailments were of a supernatural origin. To achieve balance, certain humans were granted the gift to heal. Curanderas/os are those gifted healers.

Philosophy

Curanderismo is derived from the Spanish word *curar* meaning "to heal." It is believed that the ability to heal, also called a *don* or "gift," comes from a supernatural force, and is often passed down through generations. Traditionally, healers in Curanderismo are called curanderas (females) or curanderos (males).

Curanderismo consists of various traditional healing modalities used to treat mental, physical, spiritual, and emotional maladies. It is believed that illness occurs when one (or more) of these aspects of the self are out of balance or impacted by spiritual forces. Curanderismo healing modalities stem from various cultures, civilizations, and religions, including but not limited to Aztecan, Mayan, Native American, Catholic, homeopathic, and European forms of health.

Prayer, ritual, spirituality, and connection with nature are some of the foundations of Curanderismo. Before and during healing sessions, many curanderas/os will call on support from the ancestors, the four directions, the four elements, healing tools derived from the earth, and spiritual artifacts. Altars, sacred spaces for connecting to spirit or making offerings or sacrifices, are often found in the home of curanderas/os, serving as spiritual centerpieces to ground them into their healing work.

Depending upon the person, the curandera/o may have any number of specialty areas; for example, working with herbs (*yerberas*); conducting midwifery (*parteras*); healing sprained muscles (*sobadoras*); or performing prayer (*oracionistas*), aromatherapy, or massage. A curandera-total is a healer who can work in all of the above areas and, because of this, is a highly regarded healer.

In the past, a curandera/o within a community may have lived solely on offerings from the community given in gratitude for healings. Present day curanderas/os may charge fees for their services and often have other sources of income to supplement living expenses.

Practices: What to Expect

Since Curanderismo healing specialties and the ailments being treated vary widely with each curandera/o and client, treatment can look very different and can include a variety of modalities.

Often, a curandera/o may begin with a *plática* (heart-to-heart conversation) to learn more about the experiences of the client and the client's reasons for seeking healing. Typically, prior to commencing any healing work, a sacred space is created by cleansing the room (this may be done before the client arrives) and the client with the smoke of sacred plants like dried sage, copal, or palo santo. During this time, the healer calls for support from the ancestors and Mother Earth to assist with the healing.

Some examples of what may occur during a healing include prayer, *limpia* (a spiritual cleansing method often using an egg or herbs), sound healing (using chanting or tools such as conch shells), massage, guided imagery, prescribing of herbs, energy cleanses, and *bajos* (herbal vaginal steam baths). Clients are often alone with the curandera/o and possibly his or her apprentice, but clients can be seen as a couple or group if the situation calls for it.

Setting: Home or community settings.
Duration: 1–2 hours.
Cost: From bartered goods to $150.

Best Suited for These Conditions

- Alcoholism
- Allergies
- Anxiety
- Asthma
- Back pain
- Bacterial infections
- Chronic non-malignant pain
- Depression
- Diabetes
- Emotional difficulties
- Fatigue
- Financial difficulties
- Headaches
- Impotence/Infertility
- Indigestion
- Maternity care and delivery
- Psychiatric disorders
- Social problems
- Trauma

Coaching Tip

Due to the deeply cultural nature of this form of healing, it is not advisable to recommend Curanderismo to clients who are unfamiliar with the practice or skeptical of it. For clients who have already had experience with or exposure to the system of Curanderismo, the coach should understand that this form of healing can be used effectively in conjunction with health coaching to support some of the spiritual work that may have been performed or suggested by a curandera/o.

Contraindication

Each modality used by the curandera/o has special considerations. For instance, when using herbs for healing, the individual contraindications for each herb should apply. Also, clients should believe in the philosophy of Curanderismo in order to effectively receive full benefits from treatment.

Research and Benefits

Currently, there is not much academic research with supported evidence of the positive effects of Curanderismo. Many of the studies conducted have included few (less than ten) participants and have seen inconclusive results. There are, however, many anecdotal reports of the benefits of Curanderismo.

Much of the current research available on Curanderismo focuses on identifying both practicing curanderas/os in the United States and their particular forms of practice. There is also ample research on the belief that Latinx populations have regarding the success of Curanderismo as a healing practice. This research shows the treatment options preferred by the Latinx population, as many people use a combination of western medicine and Curanderismo for healing.

Practitioner Training and Credentials

Many curanderas/os are born into family lineages of healers where information is passed down to the next generation. For those who are born into lineages of curanderas/os, and for those who were not but who hold spiritual gifts, there is often an apprenticeship required before one can be recognized and fully honored as a healer in the community. Apprenticeships can last many years and must be under the guidance of an experienced curandera/o. It is important to note that the healing talents the curanderas/os possess and utilize cannot be learned by anyone. There must be a spiritual calling to this work.

Resources

Books

Elena Avila. *Woman Who Glows in the Dark: A Curandera Reveals Traditional Aztec Secrets of Physical and Spiritual Health.* J. P. Tarcher/Putnam, 1999.

Robert Trotter. *Curanderismo: Mexican-American Folk Healing.* University of Georgia Press, 1981.

Websites

Center for Traditional Medicine—centerfortraditionalmedicine.org.

References

Avila, E. *Woman Who Glows in the Dark: A Curandera Reveals Traditional Aztec Secrets of Physical and Spiritual Health.* JP Tarcher/Putnam, 1999.

Brown, S. "Considering Curanderismo: The Place of Traditional Hispanic Folk Healing in Modern Medicine." 2008 bc.edu/clubs/mendel/ethos/archives/2008/brown.shtml. Accessed April 2017

Gale Encyclopedia of Alternative Medicine. April 1, 2017. As cited in encyclopedia.com. Accessed April 2017

Kennedy, L, et al. "The Effect of Curanderismo on Chronic Non-malignant Pain: A Case Report." *Explore: The Journal of Science & Healing* 12, no. 4 (July-August 2016): 263-267. doi: 10.1016/j.explore.2016.04.006.

Maduro, R. "Curanderismo and Latino Views of Disease and Curing."
    Western Journal of Medicine 139, no. 6 (1983): 868-874.
Ortiz, FM. "History of Midwifery in New Mexico: Partnership Between
    Curandera-parteras and the New Mexico Department of Health." *The
    Journal of Midwifery & Women's Health* 50 (2005): 411-417. doi:
    10.1016/j.jmwh.2004.12.001.
Padilla R, et al. "Use of Curanderismo in a Public Health Care System."
    JAMA Internal Medicine 161, no. 10 (2001): 1336-1340. doi:
    10.1001/archinte.161.10.1336.
Romero, CD, et al. "Antibacterial Properties of Common Herbal Remedies
    of the Southwest." *Journal of Ethnopharmacology* 99, no. 2 (2005):
    253-257.
Tafur, MM, et al. "A Review of Curanderismo and Healing Practices
    among Mexicans and Mexican Americans." *Occupational Therapy
    International* 16, no. 1 (2009): 82-88.
Trotter, RT & Juan Antonio Chavira. *Curanderismo: Mexican American
    Folk Healing.* University of Georgia Press, 1997.
Trotter, R. "Curanderismo: A Picture of Mexican-American Folk Healing."
    The Journal of Alternative and Complementary Medicine 7, no. 2
    (2001): 129-131.

ECOTHERAPY
Sakura Okamura

An emerging and growing field of holistic therapy that eases stress and enhances vitality through contact with nature.

History

It has long been recognized that nature has enormous healing potential, but the idea of ecopsychology did not arise in the United States until the 1990s. Ecotherapy was first named in 1996 by minister and pastoral counselor Howard Clinebell. The need for nature in our era has become urgent as we spend more time indoors and as more and more people live in cities. Author and journalist Richard Louv asserts that health issues of people, especially children, in modern society develop as a result of a deficiency of connection with nature. In 2005, Louv named the condition *nature deficit disorder*. Now as the benefits of ecotherapy are becoming well known, a wide range of clinicians incorporate ecotherapy into their practices.

Philosophy

Ecotherapy is distinct from other healthcare modalities in that it concerns not only human health, but also ecology; other healthcare modalities focus mainly on the former. This perspective is predominantly affected by the idea of *deep ecology*, which regards human beings as a part of an ecosystem, and which was developed by philosopher Arne Naess during the 1970s. Naess named the self-consciousness that integrates the self with the environment *ecological self*. Activist and author Joanna Macy called it *greening of the self*. In clinical settings, therapists do not use these terms to encourage their clients to embody the philosophy, but to emphasize reconnection with nature for clients' sustainable and optimal health.

Practices: What to Expect

Ecotherapy can take different forms. Among these forms are practices that are conducted outside and have the most direct interaction with nature. The intensity of the practices and the costs involved can vary from thirty minutes of outdoor counseling to backpacking wilderness therapy during which therapists and clients go off on adventures. One of the most common forms of outdoor ecotherapy is a guided stroll in the forest called forest bathing, also known as shinrin-yoku, which originated in Japan in 1982. Indoor meditation, guided imagery associated with nature, and practices which utilize nature images and objects are also considered forms of ecotherapy. Such practices can be combined with other modalities, including psychotherapy, as well as additional outdoor sessions. In addition to ecotherapy practices, ecotherapeutic sessions have been accepted in corporate workplaces, hospitals, clinics, schools and residential environments

Best Suited for These Conditions

Every single person can benefit from ecotherapy, regardless of one's health status, because it lowers stress levels and increases revitalization. Therefore, this modality is suitable for most mental health issues and stress-related chronic health conditions. Below is a list of conditions in which ecotherapy is likely to be applied.

- Anxiety disorder
- Depression
- Hypertension
- Mood disorder
- PTSD

Coaching Tip

Before you use any images of nature or go outside with your patients, ask them if they have had any traumatic experiences that are associated with a certain nature setting or any specific phobia. For example, if an individual has experienced tsunami in the past, showing an image of a wave in the ocean or going to a beach might trigger a flashback

Contraindications

- Psychoses
- Dissociative mental states
- Agoraphobia

Research and Benefits

When you are in the forest, you benefit from an aroma, *phytoncides*, from the trees. The forest sound has a higher vibration compared to the sounds in the city. These factors contribute to an increase in natural killer cells in your body, and a decrease in stress levels. Consequently, being in nature enhances the immune system, and relieves any stress-related symptoms or diseases, such as sleeping disorders and high blood pressure. Some counselors report that as nature becomes a witness and gives a variety of metaphors, outdoor sessions help clients become open and explore their emotions.

There are still abundant benefits from nature even if you stay indoors. Hospitalized patients who have a view of nature from their rooms can recover more quickly from their conditions. Furthermore, simply seeing nature images increases the brain's serotonin levels, dopamine, and alpha waves, all of which are associated with stress reduction. One of the ongoing researches related to ecotherapy is the effect of greening the environment. Recent studies have shown that greening the indoor environment and landscape can improve physical and mental functions as well as ease stress levels.

Practitioner Training and Credentials
Forest Therapy Guide Training by the Association of Nature & Forest Therapy
(natureandforesttherapy.org/guide-training-overview.html)
TerraSoma Ecopsychology Training Institute in California
(wildernessreflections.com/terrasoma-ecopsychology-training-institute)
Master program in Ecotherapy at Prescott College
(prescott.edu/academics/concentrations/ecotherapy)
Master program in Ecopsychology at Naropa University
(naropa.edu/academics/masters/ecopsychology/index.php)

Resources
Association of Nature & Forest Therapy—natureandforesttherapy.org
Sinrin-yoku—shinrin-yoku.org
Wilderness Reflections in California—wildernessreflections.com

References
Buzzel, L & Chalquist, C. *Ecotherapy: Healing with Nature In Mind.* Sierra Club Books, 2009.
Clinibell, H. Ecotherapy: Healing Ourselves, Healing the Earth. Haworth Press, 1996.
Hasbach, P & Kahn, P, editors. Ecopsychology: Science, Totems, and the Technological Species. MIT Press, 2012.
Hinds, J & Jordan, M. *Ecotherapy: Theory, Research and Practice.* Palgrave, 2016.
Louv, R. *Last Child in the Woods.* Algonquin Books, 2005.
Roszak, T, et al., editors. *Ecopsychology: Restoring the Earth, Healing the Mind.* Sierra Club Books, 1995.
Seaward, B. *Managing Stress.* 8th ed., Jones and Bartlett, 2015.

EMDR—EYE MOVEMENT DESENSITIZATION AND REPROCESSING
Emilie Miller

Eye movement desensitization and reprocessing (EMDR) is a psychotherapeutic treatment for dampening or relieving traumatic memories.

History

EMDR was developed in early 1987 by Francine Shapiro, PhD, an American psychologist. Dr. Shapiro observed, first on herself, that when moving the eyes bilaterally, from right to left and from left to right, that distressing and traumatic memories were dampened down but not suppressed. The memories were still present, but no longer had a distracting (or in some cases, profoundly disturbing) effect on the person/patient recalling them.

Shapiro's PhD dissertation was devoted to her findings, and her thesis, "Efficacy of the Eye Movement Desensitization Procedure in the Treatment of Traumatic Memories," was subsequently published in the *Journal of Traumatic Stress* in 1989. Shapiro founded the EMDR Institute, Inc., where she serves as executive director. As of 2017, Dr. Shapiro is a senior research fellow, emeritus at the Mental Research Institute in Palo Alto, CA.

EMDR is one of three treatments used by the Department of Defense in treating soldiers with post-traumatic stress disorder (PTSD) (Shapiro). The American Psychiatric Association also deems EMDR an effective treatment for those with traumatic memories, as does the International Society for Traumatic Stress Studies (Rodriguez).

Philosophy

EMDR uses bilateral stimulation with patients who are afflicted with intrusive, traumatic memories. It touches on various principles of psychotherapeutic approaches, such as behavioral, bio-informational, cognitive, family systems, somatic, and psychodynamic. The bilateral stimulation has evolved from bilateral movement of the eyes to bilateral stimulation via sound and/or tapping (Shapiro). This side-to-side repetition affects the amygdala portion of the brain, where memories, including traumatic memories, are stored. The distracting nature of the bilateral stimulation in EMDR enables the amygdala to be accessed with less effort. By accessing the amygdala, an embedded, traumatic memory can come forward, perhaps more easily than it would during a therapeutic session that solely consisted of talk therapy.

Once a memory has been recalled by the patient via bilateral stimulation, the patient is to stay present with the memory, as well as the feelings the memory brings up. Shapiro and those practicing EMDR find that if the patient is able to stay present with the memory and associated feelings, rather than dissociating or repressing, then the memory will subside, losing its power, and the feelings it brings up will decrease in intensity, becoming, while still present, now bearable.

Treatments: What to Expect

Any practitioner administering EMDR should not only be trained in EMDR, but also have training in working with those with trauma. At the end of this section are resources to assist in locating an experienced, trained EMDR specialist. If a client seeking EMDR has a current history of dissociating, resolving that symptom will become a priority before beginning with a series of EMDR treatments. Dissociating can interfere with, or even null, the effects of EMDR.

It is important that the client feel comfortable and safe with the EMDR practitioner. EMDR should not be forced upon an individual. The success of EMDR therapy relies to a great extent on the client's openness to it. Clients should always participate of their own free will.

Course of Treatment: EMDR is done in eight phases. What follows is a summation of the eight phases as described by the EMDR Institute, Inc.

In the first phase, the client's background and history are determined by the therapist. The therapist identifies where in the client's life EMDR processing will be useful. The therapist also assesses the client's ability to handle emotional distress as well as the client's readiness for therapy.

In the second phase, self-regulating techniques are established to help the client in the event that the EMDR work becomes distressing or overwhelming.

In phase three through six, the client and therapist engage in bilateral stimulation. Again, this can be via eye movement, taps, or sounds. Before the bilateral stimulation begins, the client identifies a positive belief he or she has. During the bilateral stimulation, the client recalls a visual associated with the traumatic memory, a negative belief, and a sensation within the body related to the memory and belief. The length of time during which the bilateral stimulation occurs depends on the client. Should the client dissociate, the stimulation ends.

During these three phases, the client and therapist are working, via the bilateral stimulation, to reduce the amount of distress associated with the memory. Being in tune with the feelings in the body helps measure the distress level. Once there is no distress associated with the memory, the client, guided by the therapist, begins to focus on the aforementioned positive belief, which is a resource to draw upon should the client be faced with future distress or a triggering situation.

In phase seven, the client keeps a log which tracks life events, including those that are distressing, and how the client chooses to self-sooth and manage his or her emotions.

In phase eight, the progress made in the previous seven phases is examined and discussed. Based on what arises in phase eight, the client and therapist choose how best to proceed therapeutically.

Setting: Seated comfortably in a non-threatening room.
Duration: 60–90 minutes.
Cost: $100–350

Best Suited for These Conditions

EMDR is most widely used and recognized for the treatment of:

- PTSD
- C-PTSD (complex post-traumatic stress disorder—multiple traumas)
- It has also been shown to be effective for the following:
- Traumatic memories
- Psychological trauma
- Emotional abuse
- Physical abuse
- Sexual assault (recent or past)
- Addiction
- Stress and anxiety reduction

There is anecdotal support that suggests that EMDR may be helped in treating panic disorders, dissociative disorders, phobias, anxiety surrounding public speaking, body dysmorphic disorder, depression, and attachment disorder.

Coaching Tip

If any of your clients are interested in EMDR, recommend that they also work with a mental health counselor or psychotherapist in order to process any trauma or troubling memories.

Contraindications

EMDR will bring up distressing memories. Before beginning the reprocessing, the purpose of the pre-determined, client-established, self-soothing techniques is to preempt any fear or lack of control brought up by the distressing memories and to bring the client back to being and feeling safe.

Both extreme emotions and physical responses may occur for the client during the EMDR session. A well-trained EMDR therapist will know how to handle such a situation and guide the client to safety. This is why the feeling of safety in the setting of the session is so imperative. Once the client believes that there is no threat being posed, the visuals, scents, and atmosphere of the therapeutic setting must further instill safety and wellbeing.

EMDR is not recommended for pregnant women or those prone to seizures. It is important for the client to provide the EMDR therapist with a list of any medications and/or supplements being taken. Those with dissociative disorder are not encouraged to partake in EMDR treatments, as fully confronting the memories brought up in EMDR is essential to its effectiveness, and therefore its ability to provide relief and recovery.

Research and Benefits

A study conducted by the Cochrane Common Mental Disorders Group on the effects of psychological treatments in cases of PTSD, published first in 2005 and then updated in 2007 and in 2013, states in its findings that "EMDR did better than waitlist/usual care in reducing clinician-assessed PTSD symptoms" (Andrew).

Bessel van der Kolk, MD, a foremost researcher on PTSD, C-PTSD, and the effects psychological and physical trauma have on children and adults, founded and operates The Trauma Clinic in Boston, MA. Van der Kolk has been one of the pioneers in expanding beyond talk therapy to treat traumatized individuals. Studying both the brain and body, van der Kolk holds yearly conferences bringing together trauma researchers and clinicians to discuss the mysterious and insidious ways in which trauma affects one's constitution.

In his own practice, van der Kolk utilizes EMDR therapy with his patients due to the successful results he has witnessed among patients under his care, and those being treated by his colleagues. In his first experience administering EMDR, van der Kolk was struck by the fact that he was treating a traumatized individual yet engaging in very little, if any, talk therapy. He also made note of the marked juxtaposition between the client's highly emotional state upon beginning the treatment and the client's ultimate relaxation at the end of the EMDR session (van der Kolk). Afterward, van der Kolk noted that EMDR is indeed able to help clients quickly access the (painful) memories from their past. Accessing them and confronting them seemed to put the experiences "into a larger context or perspective" (van der Kolk). Van der Kolk also saw that it was possible, if not more effective, for those with trauma to heal from it without talking about it. Van der Kolk noted that EMDR appeared "to cure some of the patients whom he'd been unable to help before" (van der Kolk).

Encouraged by the success EMDR was having on his patients, in 2007 he and his colleagues led a study funded by the National Institute of Mental Health in which they compared the results of EMDR on people with PTSD with those of Prozac and a placebo. There were eighty-eight subjects. Of them, thirty received EMDR, twenty-eight were given Prozac, and the remainder were given the placebo. The study was eight weeks in length, with those receiving EMDR improving significantly over those taking Prozac or the placebo. Van der Kolk and his colleagues found that one in four of those receiving EMDR were "completely cured" (van der Kolk). He stressed that the true signifier of the effectiveness of EMDR came in looking at the long-term effects. Eight months after the study had ended, van der Kolk found that of those who received EMDR, 60 percent tested as cured.

Practitioner Training and Credentials

In looking for an EMDR clinician/therapist or practitioner, it is first important to look for someone who has at least a few years of experience in EMDR. This will not only help the client by eliminating choices, but also improve the client's chance of eventual success with his or her chosen EMDR therapist. Being under the care of a seasoned, confident professional will also help create safety for the client.

The EMDR International Association (EMDRIA) is based in Austin, TX, with certified practitioners all over the world. All EMDRIA practitioner candidates have been licensed or certified in additional therapeutic modalities, which they have been practicing professionally for at least two years. The EMDRIA training in EMDR includes 50 clinical sessions of EMDR and twenty-four hours of EMDR consultation with an EMDR-approved consultant. Those certified by EMDRIA must complete continuing education courses every two years to keep their certification current and in good standing (emdria.org).

The EMDR Institute, Inc. is run by Dr. Francine Shapiro. Her certification program is designed for licensed mental health professionals seeking to expand therapeutic devices and offerings to their clients. The certification takes place over two weekends, includes outside reading, and ten hours of case consultation with an EMDR approved consultant. There are five months between the first and second weekend of the training. During this time, the case consultation takes place. Continuing education and advanced specialty workshops are offered to those who have completed the certification (emdr.com).

Resources

EMDR Institute, Inc[*]—emdr.com.

EMDR International Association (EMDRIA)[*]—emdria.org.

EMDR-Therapy[*]—emdr-therapy.com/emdr.htm.

The International Society of Traumatic Stress Studies—istss.org.

Trauma Recovery: EMDR Humanitarian Assistance Programs
     emdrhap.org.

* Note: These organizations offer information on EMDR, assistance in locating an
     EMDR clinician, and information on EMDR training for professionals.

References

Andrew, M, et al. "Psychological Therapies for Chronic Post-Traumatic
     Stress Disorder (PTSD) in Adults." *The Cochrane Database of
     Systematic Reviews*, 2013, doi: 10.1002/14651858.CD003388.pub4.
     Accessed April, 2017.

The EMDRIA Family of Sites. The EMDR International Association,
     emdria.org. Accessed March and April, 2017.

The EMDR Institute, Inc. Family of Sites. The EMDR Institute, Inc.,
     emdr.com. Accessed April, 2017.

"EMDR with Dr. Blanche Freund." *The Experts Speak* from An
     Educational Service of the Florida Psychiatric Society, April 7, 2014,
     katenagroup.org/expertsspeak/BLANCHE_FREUND_PHD_EMDR_A
     PRIL2014.mp3. Accessed April, 2017.

"Getting Past Your Past with Francine Shapiro." *Strategies for Living* from
     David McMillian, 6 July 2012.
     strategiesforliving.com/podcast.php?p=2194. Accessed April, 2017.

Rodriguez, T. "Can Eye Movements Treat Trauma?" Scientific American,
     1 January 2013. scientificamerican.com/article/can-eye-movements-
     treat-trauma/?page=1. Accessed April, 2017.

Shapiro, F. *Getting Past Your Past: Take Control of Your Life with Self-
     Help Techniques from EMDR Therapy*. Rodale, 2012.

van der Kolk, B. *The Body Keeps the Score*. Penguin Books, 2014.

FASTING
Elaine Santos

A fast is a practice that can mean abstaining completely from food or abstaining from or consuming only specific foods or beverages (for example, a juice fast). Fasts can last from twelve hours to weeks or months.

History

Fasting is an ancient religious, spiritual, and health practice that is used to this day. Historically, Hippocrates and Plutarch are examples of medical people who promoted fasting as a health cure. Other notable pioneers of medicine and science have advocated fasting, such as Swiss German physician Paracelsus (1493–1541) and Benjamin Franklin (1706–1790). In the 1900s, an article on therapeutic fasting as a safe and effective way to lose weight was published in the *Journal of Biological Chemistry*. The 1950s and 1960s saw more interest in the medical community in therapeutic fasting, but it faded from the mainstream by the 1980s (Fung & Moore, 67–68).

In recent years, the 5:2 Diet has popularized intermittent fasting. Intermittent fasting is creating an eating and fasting schedule. The 5:2 Diet, as an example, is five days of normal eating and then two days of fasting (O'Connor). Other intermittent fasting schedules are 16 hours of fasting and 8 hours of eating in one day. Intermittent fasting schedules are flexible to the individual, and beverages such as non-sweetened tea and coffee are allowed on fasting days (along with water).

Philosophy

In traditional cultures, a natural cycle of feast and famine, as well as specific fasts used for healing, was common (Fallon, 612). The modern era brought an eating schedule of three meals a day plus snacks. This type of food availability is a new phenomenon. A break from eating is not as radical as it may sound at first.

There are multiple theories on fasting. The first is the general idea of using fasting to give the body a rest. The fast allows the body to detoxify, repair, and heal itself naturally. Paracelsus said this best: "Fasting is the greatest remedy—the physician within." There is also the philosophy that fasting can help jumpstart someone into a desired healthy lifestyle behavior change. This philosophy comes from a health clinic that conducted research on patients with hypertension. They found that participants continued the desired change to a healthier diet after supervised water fasting (healthpromoting.com/water-fasting/fasting-research).

One theory on the physiological benefits of intermittent fasting is that it causes slight stress on the cells, and then the cells adapt and potentially resist disease. This is similar to the stress caused during exercise; as long as there is recovery time, the body gets stronger (Collier).

Fasting for health isn't just about *not eating*: the kinds of foods eaten before and after a fast are important as well. It is recommended to stop consuming alcohol, refined sugar, and caffeine before fasting. Practitioners require a period before and after water fasting of eating only vegetables and juices. Practitioners advocating intermittent fasting tend to promote a high-fat, low-carb diet to help the body transition to burning fat instead of glucose.

Practices: What to Expect

The physician or practitioner will want the patient's health history, current medications, and eating habits or current diet information. There will be a pre-fasting diet and a plan, and a schedule of what type and duration fast the client will commit to (intermittent, extended, water, juice, etc.).

Symptoms such as headache and acne can occur since the body is detoxing. It is a best practice, before beginning a fast, to phase out certain foods, such as caffeine, alcohol, and refined sugar. It is equally important to add food back slowly after a fast. If on a water-only fast, symptoms of hunger usually decline after day two.

Setting: Doctor's or other practitioner's office, or health center.
Duration: Depends on condition and professional recommendation.
Cost: $120 per hour to $4,000 for entire fasting programs.

Best Suited for These Conditions

- Obesity and weight management
- Type 2 diabetes
- Digestive issues
- Some cancers

Coaching Tip

If your coaching clients are interested in fasting, and they have a chronic condition or are taking medications, you will need to request that they work with their medical doctor, or you can ask them to research a clinical practitioner who has expertise in nutrition and fasting. Since fasting can mean from one day to months of abstaining from all food, or abstaining from specific foods, you might consider exploring your client's health goals to see what type of fasting might be a good fit for them. Caution them that fasting is a powerful healing technique and that the food eaten before and after a fast are important to consider when creating the fasting plan.

Contraindications

- Fasting should not be practiced by people who are:
- Pregnant or breastfeeding
- Under eighteen years of age
- Malnourished or underweight
- Hypoglycemic
- Professional supervision or consultation is advised for people with:
- Gout
- Type 1 or Type 2 diabetes,
- Gastroesophageal reflux disease (GERD)
- Professional supervision or consultation is also advised for people taking medication.

Research and Benefits

The benefits of fasting are numerous, and research is catching up to the anecdotal evidence. There are many animal studies showing the benefits of fasting and alternate-day fasting, with a smaller but growing number of studies with human participants (Collier; Fuhrman). Research and anecdotal evidence show benefits to the following conditions:

- Weight management and obesity
- Type 2 diabetes: Fasting can boost the power of low-carbohydrate diets to lower blood sugar and can stop insulin resistance when caloric reduction doesn't
- Digestive issues
- Hypertension
- Cancer
- Mild cognitive impairment

There is new evidence pointing to potential therapeutic benefits from short, nightly twelve-hour fasts lasting from around 6 pm or dinner time to the first meal of the next day in reducing the glycotoxic effects that contribute to mild cognitive impairment, dementia and certain subtypes of early Alzheimer's disease. The Ketoflex 12/3 diet recommended by Dale Bredesen, MD (Bredesen), is part of a complex protocol that has demonstrated a reversal of cognitive decline in over 200 peer-reviewed case studies. Large multi-site trials are now ongoing. This twelve-hour intermittent fast also recommends stopping eating at least three hours before bedtime.

Practitioner Training and Credentials

People with chronic conditions or people who want to fast for extended periods of time should consult with a medical doctor. If a client does not have access to an MD who will work with them on a fast, they can also seek a naturopathic doctor (ND) or a doctor of chiropractic (DC) who has nutritional training.

There are doctors who specialize in fasting for chronic conditions at health clinics, and there is certification from the International Association of Hygienic Physicians (IAHP), a professional association for licensed primary care physicians (medical doctors, osteopaths, chiropractors, and naturopaths) who specialize in therapeutic fasting supervision as an integral part of hygienic care (iahp.net).

Resources

Intensive Dietary Management—intensivedietarymanagement.com
Whole Health MD—wholehealthmd.com
International Association of Hygienic Physicians—iahp.net
TrueNorth Health Education Center—Healthpromoting.com/water-
     fasting/fasting-research

References

Bjarnadottir, A. "The Beginner's Guide to The 5:2 Diet." authoritynutrition.com/the-5-2-diet-guide. Accessed 9 April 2017.

Bredesen, D. *The End of Alzheimer's.* Avery, 2017.

Collier, R. "Intermittent Fasting: The Science of Going Without." *CMAJ.* 85, no. 9 (June 11, 2013): E363–E364. doi: 10.1503/cmaj.109-4451 PMCID: PMC3680567.

Fallon, S & Enig, MG. *Nourishing Traditions.* Revised 2nd edition. New Trends Publishing, 1999.

Fuhrman, J. *Fasting and Eating for Health.* St. Martin's Griffin, 1995.

Fung, J & Moore, J. *The Complete Guide to Fasting.* Victory Belt Publishing, 2016.

Goldhamer, A, Lisle, D, Parpia, B, Anderson, SV, & Colin, CT. "Medically Supervised Water-only Fasting in the Treatment of Hypertension." *Journal of Manipulative and Physiological Therapeutics*, 24, no. 5 (June 2001).

O'Connor, A. "Fasting Diets Are Gaining Acceptance." well.blogs.nytimes.com/2016/03/07/intermittent-fasting-diets-are-gaining-acceptance/?_r=0. Accessed 9 April 2017.

Robinson, M. "These Silicon Valley 'biohackers' Are Fasting Their Way to Longer, Better Lives." 6 Aug 2016, businessinsider.com/silicon-valley-biohacking-wefast-2016-8/#the-first-rule-of-wefast-is-you-eat-as-soon-as-your-food-hits-the-table-1. Accessed 9 April 2017.

Varady, KA & Hellerstein, MK. "Alternate-day fasting and chronic disease prevention: a review of human and animal trials." *The American Journal of Clinical Nutrition* 86, no. 1 (July 2007). 7–13.

Weil, A. "Intermittent Fasting: A Healthy Choice." 6 June 2012. huffingtonpost.com/andrew-weil-md/fasting-health_b_1557043.html. Accessed 9 April 2017.

FLOWER ESSENCES
Brooke Griffin

Flower essences are subtle energy, vibrational remedies that work to bring balance to the mind-body connection by addressing the energetic field of the being. They can be taken internally or applied externally.

History

Flower essences were first popularized in the 1930s by Dr. Edward Bach, an English medical doctor and bacteriologist. He discovered these remedies by collecting dew-drops from certain plants, leaves, and branches, and then experimenting with these water drops as remedies for his patients. "Through his sensitive observation of nature and of human suffering, he was able to correlate each plant remedy with specific human states of mind" (Kaminski, 13). Dr. Bach developed a system known as Bach Flower Essences, consisting of thirty-nine remedies that he believed could address any and all conditions.

Many systems have been developed in the years since, extending beyond these thirty-nine remedies, including both single-plant remedies and combination remedies. The remedies are prepared outdoors in precise weather conditions, adding plant material to a clear glass bowl full of pure spring water. The bowl is left alone for several hours, in pure sunlight with no clouds in the sky. Some makers additionally use astrology and the phases of the moon to change the vibration of the remedies. Each plant material infuses the water with its unique vibration. The solution then is strained to remove the plant material, preserved in brandy, and diluted many times over. Much like homeopathy, there is virtually none of the plant material left in the resulting solution. The vibration of the plant's energy is what makes flower essences so special. Today, flower essences can be found in almost any health food store, natural pharmacy, or apothecary, and are quite popular throughout Europe.

Philosophy

Flower essences are gentle remedies that balance the emotions by addressing the energetic field of the being, whether it is human, animal, or plant. Flower essences are most often used to address emotional states and are said to have a so-called onion peeling effect, in which the remedy chosen addresses the most current state. Flower essence therapy addresses the whole person and the person's emotions or feelings around a situation, rather than addressing a disease itself. Flower essence therapy has been called "soul therapy through flower energy" (Scheffer, 10).

"As Bach explained in his landmark treatise *Heal Thyself*, disease is a message to change, an opportunity to become aware of our shortcoming and to learn the lessons of life experience so that we may better fulfill our true destiny" (Kaminski, 12-13).

Treatments: What to Expect

Flower essence therapy is typically conducted as a consultation during which the clients explain what it is they would like to work on, adjust, change, or shift, or what is present in their lives and how they emotionally relate to the topic or concern. The practitioner is not a psychotherapist and does not analyze or offer advice. The practitioner listens and educates the client regarding remedies that may address the particular emotions the client has expressed. The practitioner will go over the selected remedies with the client and explain how often to take them. Up to seven essences can be combined at one time. Although the remedies are most often taken internally because they are simply vibration, they can be used topically just as effectively, making them safe for alcoholics in recovery, babies, the elderly, and animals. A mantra or positive affirmation is often given to say along with the remedy each time it is taken.

Setting: private consultation office.
Duration: ~60 minutes.
Cost: ~$60.

Best Suited for These Conditions

- Stress
- Emergencies
- Psychosomatic issues
- Emotional states
- Spiritual issues
- Trauma recovery
- Loss, grief, or bereavement
- Personality imbalances
- Addictions
- Sleep disorders
- Flower essences may also be helpful with
- Changing patterns
- Patients in hospice and the terminally ill
- Personal transformation and growth

Flower essences are useful and safe for animals and plants.

Coaching Tip

You cannot go wrong by offering this approach to your client. It is gentle and non-invasive. Even if the wrong remedy is chosen, there are no dangerous side effects; the remedy will simply not have any effect. Finding a practitioner who can work with the client to understand the client's most present emotions or state is important in the process of choosing the correct remedy. Encourage your client to speak to the flower essence practitioner about present-moment emotions or states regarding the topic of concern, without focusing on emotions that are not presently relevant in the moment of the consultation.

Contraindications

There are no known contraindications. Flower essences are safe to use with other modalities and medications under the care of a physician. The remedies are made in an alcohol base, usually brandy, so be aware of this in the condition of alcoholism and recommend that the remedy be applied topically rather than taken internally.

Research and Benefits

First-hand reports show the effectiveness of flower essence therapy in bringing balance to emotional states. Although there is very little scientific research available to back this, some research is available. In 2007, a double-blind clinical trial was conducted on individuals with acute situational stress using a standard dose of the Bach Flower Essence's *Rescue Remedy* and a placebo with the control group. The results showed that Rescue Remedy may be effective in reducing high levels of situational anxiety (Halberstein). Another research study showed positive results when flower essences were used as a placebo in conjunction with a positive therapeutic ritual (Hyland).

Flower essences are often accompanied with a positive affirmation, and another research study shows that the affirmation enhances the effectiveness of the remedy. Flower essences are vibrational remedies that address the emotions, and affirmations impact the vibration and emotional states as well.

Flower essences are known to be safe and gentle, making them a fantastic remedy for all, including the elderly, children, pets, and even plants. There are many progressive veterinary clinics and animal shelters that use flower essences with the animals to help them recover from trauma and to calm their nervous systems.

Practitioner Training and Credentials

There is no governing body that regulates the training or certification of flower essence practitioners. Training programs are determined by the specific companies that have training schools, such as the Bach Foundation and Flower Essences Society. Additionally, flower essence training is often included in the curricula of herbal schools and naturopathic schools. Although the Bach Foundation is based in England, they offer three levels of training throughout the world. Level 1 is available both in-person and through distance training. Levels 2 and 3 must be completed in person. There is ongoing support from the Bach Foundation for their registered practitioners, such as training and practice materials. Materials are provided if the practitioner would like to perform demonstrations.

Resources
Alaskan Essences—alaskanessences.com
Bach Flower Essences—bachflower.com
Flower Essence Services (FES)—fesflowers.com
Perelandra Essences—perelandra-ltd.com

References
Kaminski, Pa & Katz, R. *Flower Essence Repertory.* Earth-Spirit, Inc. 1996.
Halberstein, R, DeSantis, L, Sirkin, A, Padron-Fajardo, V, & Ojeda-Vaz, M. "Healing with Bach Flower Essences: Testing a Complimentary Therapy." journals.sagepub.com/doi/pdf/10.1177/1533210107300705
Hyland, M, Whalley, B, & Geraght, AWA. "Dispositional predictors of placebo responding: A motivational interpretation of flower essence and gratitude therapy." Journal of *Psychosomatic Research* 62, no. 3 (2007). 331–34. sciencedirect.com/science/article/pii/S0022399906004582
Scheffer, M. *The Encyclopedia of Bach Flower Therapy.* Healing Arts Press, 2001, pp 10.

GUIDED IMAGERY
Julie Viellieu

Guided imagery is the use of image-rich words and sounds clustered around a theme that evokes emotions appropriate to creating new neural pathways in order to bring about an intentional change in behavior of mind, body, and/or emotions (Davenport).

History

For most of history, nearly every culture has embraced a holistic view, regarding life as an interaction among body, mind, and spirit. Ancient cultures, like those of Egypt, Greece, China, India, and Tibet, as well as most indigenous cultures, had rich traditions and rituals that recognized and fostered the body-mind-spirit interconnection to promote healing and transformation. In these holistic practices, imagery naturally flourished and was an integral part of most oral traditions and religions. When literacy rates were very low and books were scarce, the use of images, symbols, and the oral tradition became the most efficient and powerful methods to pass down complex metaphysical and existential concepts (Davenport).

Philosophy

Ancient medicine is rich in imagery, and almost every culture has used religious imagery as part of its healing rites. In these cultures, images of body, mind, and spirit, and of the interactions between spirituality and health, were an integral part of daily life. In both Eastern and Western cultures, imagery and guided imagery were not practices that occurred in isolation or during scheduled sessions; rather, they were part of the dominant worldview essential for understanding and interacting with this world and the next (Davenport).

Practices: What to Expect

Guided imagery can have significant therapeutic effects within a wide range of medical applications. Guided imagery practitioners evoke or suggest mental imagery to gain diagnostic information, help people better understand themselves, and positively influence psychology and physiology.

Setting: Professional or home setting, or by phone, either individually or group.

Duration: Duration varies, but usually under one hour.

Cost: $50–150.

Best Suited for These Conditions

- Chronic pain
- Acute pain
- Sleep disorders
- Allergies
- Asthma
- Fertility
- Childbirth
- Anxiety
- Depression
- Stress
- Cancer
- Preparing for or recovering from surgery

Coaching Tip

Coaches should obtain specialized training and certification in guided imagery. Guiding people on an inward journey is a significant responsibility. Consider recommending to your clients that they work with a certified guided imagery therapist if you are unsure of the methodology. When working with a client who is undergoing a life transition (move, career, divorce, illness, etc.), it is helpful to introduce guided imagery for greater presence of mind, balance, and coping skills. Coaches might also use guided imagery whenever the client needs to tap into enhanced creativity for solving problems or devising a more effective or enjoyable way to reach goals. Ensure that there is sufficient time in the coaching session for the client to come out of the deeply relaxed state of mind, become grounded, and be able to reflect on what was discovered during the guided imagery session.

Contraindications

Guided imagery is not recommended for patients with paranoid schizophrenia.

Guided imagery should not be imposed on anyone who is made more anxious by having to sit still and relax.

Caution should be exercised when working with trauma survivors, given that some may be flooded with anxiety when imagery is introduced.

Some people may be challenged and even overwhelmed by imaginative efforts and judgment should be exercised before employing techniques like guided imagery.

Patients with hearing deficits may be frustrated by guided imagery, especially elderly patients with hearing loss in the lower registers who may not be able to hear the narrative.

Research and Benefits

Guided imagery is becoming more accepted as mainstream medicine embraces the technique as a convenient, low cost, and effective intervention (Leviton). Imagery has a variety of benefits including reducing stress, developing self-esteem and self-worth, enhancing concentration, healing trauma, minimizing pain, overcoming fears and anxiety, and dealing with grief (Davenport). There are no side effects of guided imagery; however, certified practitioners are advised to be aware that imagery may trigger a previous trauma with individuals who come from a traumatic background (Davenport). Patients with a history of mental illness, or those who have trouble distinguishing the real world from the imaginary world, must proceed with caution.

Guided imagery is effective in any age group and may be done one-on-one or in a group setting. Rappaport suggests the best practice for children and adolescents is the use of guided imagery in conjunction with focusing-orientated art therapy. After a guided imagery session, art materials are provided to the child or adolescent to encourage reflection. A patient may draw, color, or write in a journal to create art to express the feelings encountered in the guided imagery session (Rappaport).

Benefits are:

- Improved clarity in life
- Spiritual development
- Elation, freedom, and expanded awareness
- Emotional and physical healing
- Enhanced creativity
- Profoundly deep relaxation
- Increased confidence and personal empowerment
- An opening of the heart and healing of relationships
- Curing of negativity or self-defeating behaviors
- Improved performance in business or sports
- Resolution of psychological difficulties

Resources

Alchemy of the Heart—lesliedavenport.com
Healing Journeys, Belleruth Naparstek—healthjourneys.com/Belleruth
Martin Rossman, *Guided Imagery for Self-Healing*—thehealingmind.com

References

Davenport, L. *Cultivating the Imagination for Healing, Change, and Growth Transformative Imagery*. Jessica Kingsley Publishers, 2016.

Leviton, C & P. Leviton. What is Guided Imagery? The Cutting-Edge Process in Mind/Body Medical Procedures. *Annals of the American Psychotherapy Association* 7, no.2 (2004), 22-29.

Rappaport, L. *Focusing-Oriented Art Therapy Accessing the Body's Wisdom and Creative Intelligence.* Jessica KingsleyPublishers (2009).

The Benefits of Guided Meditation. (n.d.). the-guided-meditation-site.com/benefits-of-guided-meditation.html. Accessed April 18, 2017.

HERBALISM (WESTERN)
Christine Leonard

In every culture throughout the world you will find a great body of folklore concerning the indigenous plants of that region and the wise women who used them.

—Rosemary Gladstar

Hundreds of plant species serve as important sources of medicine used in modern and traditional healthcare systems around the world.

—Stephen Foster

Herbalism is the practice of treating and preventing a spectrum of conditions in all people of all ages with plant medicines prepared a variety of ways. Herbalism has roots in cultural traditions all over the world.

History
For thousands of years, cultures all over the globe have tended, gathered, and prepared plants as medicine. When the new tradition of allopathic medicine emerged in the United States, herbalism fell by the wayside because it was seen as primitive and illegitimate. However, many indigenous cultures were not dislocated from their rooted connection with plants. As natural remedies become more popular in today's modern culture in the US, herbalism is again visible to the masses. Rosemary Gladstar writes, "Working in concert, allopathic medicine and herbalism can enhance our possibilities for wellbeing." (Gladstar)

Today, Western herbalism is regaining a place of recognition as a healing modality. There is still much skepticism and attacks on the efficacy of herbs as medicine. The scientific community attempts to analyze the constituents of herbs with the shortcomings of the scientific method. Plants have some consistency among species, but the growing conditions, weather, soil content, rainfall, elevation, and numerous other factors affect the concentration and expression of constituents, giving plants a spectral concentration and consistency.

Philosophy
"Western herbal medicine is based upon a body of knowledge and experience that has as much clinical value as any other medicine." (Hoffman) Many people in the United States today study herbalism under indigenous teachers or mentors, as well as under some commonly known published herbalists. All herbalists have their own lineage of knowledge and their own approach to the client.

Allopathic medicine provides symptomatic relief, while the use of herbs as medicine provide lasting change at the root cause of the symptom. The practice of food and herbs as medicine comes into play with the use of culinary spices and may begin with the addition of black pepper to your morning egg. Every culture and tradition of food preparation has some use of herbs and spices, and every plant has some medicinal action. Herbal medicine is foremost among traditional medicine systems around the globe. (Akerele)

Treatments: What to Expect:

An herbalist's intake process can take anywhere from a half hour to two and a half hours. There is usually an extensive intake form to complete. A session will consist of talking one-on-one about the determined ailments or concerns. The herbalist will either put together a formula at the appointment or after, for pick up. Formulas may be in the form of tinctures, teas, salves, or capsules, depending on what is being treated. There will often be dietary or lifestyle suggestions, and follow-up appointments may be necessary. Often, after the initial intake, appointments may be attended by phone, Zoom, or Skype.

Setting: Herbal retail store, private or home office.
Duration: 30–120 minutes.
Cost: $30–250.

Best Suited for These Conditions

- Immunity: cold or flu and prevention
- Hypertension and blood pressure regulation
- Thyroid—hypo- or hyper-
- Reproductive hormone imbalance
- Reproductive organ issues
- Musculoskeletal conditions
- Nerve-related conditions
- Depression, anxiety, mood regulation
- Tissue repair
- As an antibiotic, antimicrobial, antiviral, or antibacterial to treat wounds, infections, and inflammation
- Digestive upset and disorders, including acid reflux, ulcers, bile production, low HCl, CIBO, leaky gut syndrome, diarrhea, gas, bloating, constipation, and hemorrhoids
- Respiratory ailments
- Cancer treatment: related side effects
- Urinary tract and bladder infections
- Pain management

Coaching Tip

For best results, recommend that your client work with experienced or certified herbalists who understand how to crosscheck for potential interference with prescription medication, and how to detect and resolve allergic reactions.

Contraindications

Individual herbs have their own list of contraindications.

Many herbs should be used under the guidance of a professional herbalist, especially during pregnancy and lactation and when used for children and animals.

Research and Benefits

Scientific study of herbalism is fairly limited. Many articles reveal the effects of herbs on animals. The amount of research is growing. More and more research by the scientific community is available on Chinese herbs in particular. Many herbalism texts can be referenced in the databases below, revealing their properties and benefits as studied over time and tradition.

Practitioner Training and Credentials

There are many professional and clinical herbalist training schools, courses, apprenticeships, conferences, workshops, and intensives available all over the US. Herbalist certification is not a national or state certification. It is important to inquire about the credentials of the practitioner you plan to see, and find out if there are reputable sources, testimonials, or reviews. Many herbalists have had a teacher, and many do a great deal of self-study.

Resources

Herbal Resources

American Botanical Council—herbalgram.org
American Herbalist Guild—americanherbalistguild.com
Arizona Ethnobotanical Research Association—
    wintersun.com/arizonaEthnobotanicalResearchAssociation
National Center for the Preservation of Medicinal Herbs—ncpmh.org
United Plant Savers—unitedplantsavers.org

Herbal Databases

A Modern Herbal (1931, by Mrs. Maude Grieve)—
    botanical.com/botanical/mgmh/mgmh.html
Dr. Duke's Phytochemical and Ethnobotanical Database—
    phytochem.nal.usda.gov/phytochem/searchars-grin.gov/duke
Henriette's Homepage—henriettes-herb.com
Lloyd Library and Museum—lloydlibrary.org

Southwest School for Botanical Medicine—swsbm.com

Bulk herbs, herbal extracts, and herbal supplies
Mountain Rose Herbs—mountainrose herbs.com
Starwest Botanicals—starwest-botanicals.com
Pacific Botanicals—pacificbotanicals.com

Herb Books
Arvigo, Rosita, Nadine Epstein, and Marilyn Yaquinto. *Sastun: My Apprenticeship with a Maya Healer*. Harper, 1994.
Buhner, Stephen Harrod. *The Secret Teachings of Plants: The Intelligence of the Heart in the Direct Perception of Nature*. Inner Traditions/Bear & Co, 2004.
Garrett, James T. *The Cherokee Herbal: Native Plant Medicine from the Four Directions*. Inner Traditions/Bear & Co, 2003.
Gladstar, Rosemary. *Rosemary Gladstar's Family Herbal: A Guide to Living Life with Energy, Health, and Vitality*. Storey Books, 2001.
Moore, Michael. *Medicinal Plants of the Pacific West*. UNM Press, 2011.
Prechtel, Martín. *The Unlikely Peace at Cuchumaquic: The Parallel Lives of People as Plants: Keeping the Seeds Alive*. North Atlantic Books, 2012.
Weed, Susun S. *Wise Woman Herbal Healing Wise*. No. 2. Ash Tree Publishing, 1989.
Wood, Matthew. *The Practice of Traditional Western Herbalism: Basic Doctrine, Energetics, and Classification*. North Atlantic Books, 2004.

References
Akerele, O & Ayinde, BA. "Antibacterial Activities of the Volatile Oil and Aqueous Extract of Murraya Koenigii Leaves." *Nigerian Journal of Natural Products and Medicine* 2, no. 1 (1998). 44-45.
Hoffmann, D. *Medical Herbalism: The Science and Practice of Herbal Medicine*. Inner Traditions/Bear & Co, 2003.
Foster, S. *Herbal Renaissance*. Gibbs Smith 1993.
Gladstar, R. *Herbal Healing for Women*. Simon and Schuster, 1993.
Mansoor, GA. "Herbs and Alternative Therapies in the Hypertension Clinic." *American Journal of Hypertension* 14, no. 9 (2001). 971-975.
Craig, WJ. "Health-promoting properties of common herbs." *The American Journal of Clinical Nutrition* 70, no. 3 (1999). 491s–499s.

Biochemically-Based Therapies

HOMEOPATHY
Devin Hexner

Homeopathy is a form of alternative medicine that utilizes a system of targeted natural remedies (vegetable, animal, and/or mineral sources) to cure maladies.

History
In 1810, German physician, Samuel Hahnemann asserted two new medical "laws." Hahnemann called the first law *The Law of Similars*, also known as "like treats like." Hahnemann called the second law *The Law of Infinitesimals.* These two laws guided the creation of the alternative medicine known as homeopathy. Based on his studies, Hahnemann believed that substances that caused symptoms of disease could also relieve these symptoms—thus his first law. He also believed that diseases stem from issues with one's mental spirit, and with infinitesimal doses of chemical remedies, one's spirit could be activated to heal the body. An estimated five million adults and one million children use homeopathy yearly.

Philosophy
Homeopathic doctors treat patients with small doses of medicine made from plant, mineral, animal, food, and biochemical sources. Examples include arnica (plant), sulfur (mineral), calamari (food), and human growth factor (biochemical).

Homeopathic *remedies* are often distilled into sugar pellets that are placed under the tongue, but they can also be formulated into creams and gels. The ingredients of the remedies are diluted in differing amounts, which homeopathic doctors prescribe for individuals depending on their health condition.

Homeopaths evaluate an individual's *constitution* by assessing a full picture of the current health condition, personal and family history, behavior, and personality, in order to determine a specific remedy, or multiple remedies, to prescribe. Homeopaths also probe patients to describe when and where their conditions' symptoms arise (e.g., time of day, weather, etc.) to tailor the remedy. Therefore, two people who have the same diagnosis may be prescribed different remedies.

Treatments: What to Expect
Homeopaths monitor patient progress for two to six weeks, and evaluate whether the dosage or remedy needs to be changed. Patients can stop taking the remedies if symptoms subside. If symptoms persist, the

homeopath may continue the remedy, increase the dosage, or change the remedy type entirely.
Setting: Professional office.
Duration: 30–90 minutes.
Cost: $30–200.

Best Suited for These Conditions

People turn to homeopathy for an array of conditions, with some homeopaths insisting that they can help individuals with any issue, chronic or acute.

- Homeopathy is used to treat conditions like:
- Respiratory infections
- Eczema
- Irritable bowel syndrome (IBS)
- Allergies
- Arthritis
- Fatigue
- Asthma
- Migraines
- Mood disorders
- Infertility

Coaching Tip

If clients are interested in exploring homeopathy as a natural way to treat their conditions, you should make clients aware that this is not meant to be a replacement for conventional care and immunizations. While this modality has been effective for some people, there may be some risks that the FDA is monitoring due to some recent cases of negative reactions from homeopathic treatments. Reviewing the information included here, as well as consulting with various medical professionals, should be recommended before engaging in homeopathic treatments.

Contraindications

The National Institute of Health has a few notable points to consider. First, the US Food and Drug Administration (FDA) does not examine remedies for safety or effectiveness. Next, it is recommended to discuss this alternative medicine with all healthcare providers. Furthermore, homeopathy is not meant to be a replacement for conventional care and immunizations, and one should not postpone seeing a healthcare provider about medical problems.

The FDA recently discovered 400 cases of negative effects from homeopathic remedies in children over a six-year period, along with ten infant deaths; incidents included seizures, fever, shortness of breath, sleepiness, constipation, vomiting, and agitation. On September 30, 2016, the FDA officially cautioned consumers that homeopathic remedies could be harmful to children and to discontinue use.

On November 15, 2016, the Federal Trade Commission established a new enforcement regulation for homeopathic products. Since there has not been conclusive scientific evidence for the efficacy of homeopathy, over-the-counter homeopathic products must now explicitly state two things: 1) there is no scientific evidence to prove the efficacy of homeopathy; 2) that theories of homeopathy extend from the late 1700s, and are not accepted by most modern medical experts.

Research and Benefits

Since homeopathic remedies are composed of such small amounts of the specific molecules, the way homeopathic medicine may work is not fully understood. Some scientists doubt the efficacy of homeopathy, and attribute positive changes to the placebo effect. Other scientists point to certain clinical trials that may show differences between homeopathic and placebo remedies.

Studies trying to evaluate the effectiveness of homeopathy run into the issue of treatments being specifically tailored to individuals, without standard prescriptions given by homeopathic doctors; over one hundred homeopathic remedies could be prescribed for thousands of symptoms.

A meta-analysis study from 1997 published in the *Lancet* investigated one hundred randomized, placebo-controlled trials, and determined, with a 95 percent confidence interval, that clinical effects of homeopathy are not due to a placebo effect.

Practitioner Training and Credentials

Training and credentialing of homeopaths varies. Homeopathic doctors are often licensed MDs or DOs who add homeopathic expertise to their practice. Some professionals obtain certification through the Council for Homeopathic Certification, though this is not required. Some homeopaths consider themselves consultants because they are not licensed doctors. Dana Ullman, MPH, CCH, author of *Evidence-based Homeopathic Family Medicine,* provides educational consulting services and advocacy for the profession of homeopathy.

Resources

National Center for Homeopathy—homeopathycenter.org
National Center for Complementary and Integrative Health—
    nccih.nih.gov/health/homeopathy
American Institute of Homeopathy—homeopathyusa.org

References

Abbasi, J. "Amid Reports of Infant Deaths, FTC Cracks Down on Homeopathy while FDA Investigates." *Jama* 317, no. 8 (2017): 793.

Bivins, R. *Alternative Medicine? A History.* Oxford University Press, 2007.

Dossett, ML, et al. "Homeopathy Use by US Adults: Results of a National Survey." *American Journal of Public Health* 106.4 (2016): 743–745.

"Homeopathy." *National Institutes of Health.* US Department of Health and Human Services, nccih.nih.gov/health/homeopathy. Accessed April 2018.

Zollman, C, Vickers, AJ, & Richardson, J, eds. *ABC of Complementary Medicine (2).* John Wiley & Sons, 2009

HUMOR THERAPY

Cynthia Espinoza

> *Humor is emotional chaos remembered in tranquility.*
> —James Thurber

Humor therapy is a technique that uses humor and laughter as a tool both to promote health and wellness by alleviating pain and discomfort, and to enhance one's sense of wellbeing by elevating levels of happiness and joy.

History

Laughter has been around since people discovered their ability to be ticklish. Laughter has stood the test of time. The use of humor has moved generations of people around the world and in every culture, from Europe to the Middle East, from Asia and Africa to the Americas. For example, when Greek philosophers like Plato and Aristotle noticed the healing effects of humor, they wove it into their theater and treatises (Seaward, 276; Snyder et al., 93).

However, not until recent decades has light been shed on the effectiveness of humor therapy. During the 1960s, Norman Cousins was diagnosed with a rheumatoid disorder called ankylosing spondylitis. The disease was causing his connective tissues to decay (Seaward). Upon receiving his diagnosis, Cousins decided to do research on the illness. Through his study, Cousins learned that there was a connection between the manifestation of his disease and his level of anxiety and negative feelings. He reasoned that a daily practice of experiencing more positive emotions might help to combat his disease. To test his theory and to get him through this challenging season of his life, Cousins checked into a hotel and immersed himself into a collection of humorous films and TV shows. After some time, his disease went into remission, and he returned to his home (Seaward).

Philosophy

> *Laughter is the tonic, the relief, the surcease for pain.*
> —Charlie Chaplin

Throughout the ages, the philosophy surrounding humor therapy is that healing flourishes through laughter. The Greeks saw laughter as a form of enrichment. Plato particularly thought humor "nurtured the soul" and should be utilized as a healing approach (Shelly, as cited by Seaward, 276). In 1790, a German philosopher, Immanuel Kant, credited humor as a talent that allowed people to see another perspective in any given situation (Haig, as cited by Snyder et al. 93).

There are several theories that categorize what motivates different styles of humor. The *superiority theory* suggests that this approach to humor is caused at the expense of someone else so that the people making the jokes feel better about themselves (i.e., mockery or ridicule). The *incongruity theory* holds that the unexpected union of two opposites makes a subject funny. The *release/relief theory* believes that humor can be utilized to release underlying anxieties or hateful notions. The *divinity theory* considers laughter as a treasured reward from a higher power (Seaward, 278-280). Finally, the *element of surprise* from a well-told joke may cause people to burst into laughter.

Practices: What to Expect

Humor therapy is a technique that can be used independently in small groups or alongside other medical treatments to enhance the effectiveness of healing (Wren & Norred, 150). Humor has helped individuals melt away their pain and worries in any situation.

This therapy can take shape in a variety of ways. It may look like a change in mindset or a humorous interpersonal interaction, or it may turn into a comedic product that was artfully created. There is an assortment of styles of humor—parody, satire, slapstick, absurd/nonsense humor, double entendre, black humor, irony, dry humor, quick-witted humor, puns, bathroom humor, and sarcasm (Seaward, 281–285).

There is a range of ways that individuals can personally express humor. One can share a *conventional* sense of humor, which is a type of humor that more than one person finds funny. This humor is seen as collectively laughable when expressed within a group. The *life-of-the-party* sense of humor occurs when someone brings humor into the midst of a group and elevates the mood or provides a relief from tension (Seaward, 285). A person who internalizes a lot of funny thoughts may possess a *creative* sense of humor. Such an individual is often thought of as very innovative and imaginative. However, when it comes to expressing the humor outwardly, the person may be too timid to share. Lastly, there's a *good-sport* sense of humor, possessed by individuals who can take a joke or laugh at themselves. Such people tend to be light-hearted and do not take themselves too seriously (Seaward, 285-286).

Setting: Virtually anywhere.

Duration: No time limit.

Cost: Free, or groups from $12–200.

Best Suited for These Conditions

- Depression
- Anxiety
- Cancer
- Cardiovascular disease, including strokes
- HIV
- Alzheimer's disease
- Addiction (i.e., drugs or alcoholism)

Humor therapy may also:

- Help to strengthen immunity
- Promote muscle relaxation
- Assist in opening communication
- Strengthen emotional coping

Coaching Tip

Styles of humor vary from person to person. If your clients practice humor therapy, make sure they choose something that brings them laughter. Urge them to avoid touching subjects that may be sensitive or triggering. Above all, help them create a safe space with exercises and material that they can truly enjoy.

Contraindications

The contraindications of humor therapy are quite limited. Only a small number of people are not recommended to take part in this therapy, such as:

- Chronic lung disease (Bennett)
- Individuals afraid of clowns, if clowns are present (Bennett)
- Additionally, people should be warned that humor therapy can bring about:
- Hyperventilation
- Hypertension

People should also be warned that humor therapy presents a choking hazard. Carefully watch for signs of choking or refrain from eating or drinking during humor therapy, as a choking may develop.

Research and Benefits

Humor therapy is mentally, emotionally, and physiologically stimulating. Humor secretes endorphins into the brain, making one feel happier and more able to tolerate pain, which is useful for people suffering from chronic diseases (Weisenberg, as cited by Tse, Mimi, 2). This mentally stimulating aspect of humor therapy is why it has been introduced into many medical settings to complement and enhance the healing effects of treatments that are already in place to address chronic diseases (Wren & Norred, 151).

Emotionally, humor boosts mood, self-esteem, and self-confidence, and humor promotes positive human interactions and connections. This may be the reason why humor is such a widely acceptable practice. The Cancer Treatment Center of America explains the power behind humor: "Laughter is a natural medicine. It lifts our spirits and makes us feel happy. Laughter is a contagious emotion. It can bring people together. It can help us feel alive and empowered."

Additionally, humor therapy is linked to creating an array of positive physiological reactions within the body. Depending on how often you use humor therapy, the benefits may be short term or long term. In the short term, humor appears similar to the stress response because it elevates the heart rate, respiratory capacity, and oxygen consumption (Strean, 966).

However, after coming down from a period of laughter, the body enters into a higher level of relaxed resting state (Strean, 966). Laughter also provides great levels of homeostasis. In this way, humor therapy has been shown to help balance blood pressure, aid digestion, boost body circulation, and increase oxygenation of the bloodstream (Cancer Treatment Center of America). The movement generated during laughter is said to "massage" the essential organs (Seaward, 288). Tears from laughter also rid the body of toxins (Seaward, 288).

The long-term advantage of including a generous amount of humor or laughter in your life is that its presence causes an overall fortification of the immune system. Humor and laughter aid in the releasing of neuropeptides that send messages throughout the body to defend and protect a person's immunity. This process allows the body to create "natural pain killers" (Seaward, 288; Bennett, 1997). A heightened exertion of natural killer cell activity decreases the body's susceptibility to life-threatening diseases, and reduces rates of depression among people diagnosed with cancer or HIV (Strean 966). Studies also show that humor allows the body to thrive by escalating levels of immunoglobulin A, which is an antibody made in the immune system (Berk, as cited by Tse, 2). Rates of mobile and functioning T-lymphocytes also increase during humor therapy (Snyder & Lindquist, 98). Plus, humor therapy decreases the presence of cortisol, growth hormones, and epinephrine (Berk, as cited by Tse, 2).

Practitioner Training and Credentials

Unlike other specialties, humor therapy does not require any formal training or credentials (Wren & Norred, 152). It is convenient because anyone can do it! If you can gather or come up with material that makes a person or group of people laugh, then you are practicing humor therapy.

If individuals would really like to sharpen their humor skills, they can always enroll in instructional venues like The Clown School (Wren & Norred, 152), Circus Center, or Comedy College, to name a few.

One can also become a certified laughter yoga instructor. Laughter yoga came into existence because of the Laughter Club Movement, which was established in 1995 (Laughter Yoga University). While the movement provided laughter through jokes and humor, club members found themselves stuck when they ran out of material (Kataria, 6). Instead, this practice utilized laughter as a form of exercise that is not dependent on an external subject to create humor (Mora-Ripoll, 170). Laughter yoga merges the purposeful breathing accessed in yoga with unreasonable fits of laughter. Depending on the program, certification in laughter yoga can take as little as a few days, or as long as a couple of weeks or months.

Resources

There are some cost-effective approaches and resources that may be accessible to people within the convenience of their homes or social networks. From a shift in mentality to the development of a funny product, people can apply humor therapy to their daily lives by doing the following:

- Not taking life so seriously
- Finding one thing each day that makes them laugh
- Playing with their creative thoughts and making something of them
- Developing a humor library (Seaward, 291), a collection of pictures, video clips, books, movies, etc. that make them laugh
- Nurturing their self-esteem
- Branching out to create a humor network, a group of people who make them laugh and feel happy (Seaward, 291)

Along with these ideas, there are schools, programs, and organizations that people can attend to further strengthen their ability to provide humor therapy. These are a couple of selections:

The Clown School—theclownschool.com
Circus Center—circuscenter.org
The Center for Movement Theater—thisisthecenter.com/cmt.html
Celebration Barn Theater—celebrationbarn.com
San Francisco Comedy College—sfcomedycollege.com
Laughter Yoga University—laughteryoga.org
Laughter Online University—laughteronlineuniversity.com/etrainings
Laughing Rx—laughingrx.com/14.html

References

"About Laughter Yoga—Laughter Yoga University." Laughter Yoga University. laughteryoga.org/about-laughter-yoga. Accessed April 2017.

Berk, RA. "The Active Ingredients in Humor: Psychophysiological Benefits and Risks for Older Adults." *Educational Gerontology* 27, no. 3-4 (2001): 323–339.

Bennett, M. "The Effect of Mirthful Laughter on Stress and Natural Killer Cell Cytotoxicity." Effect of Mirthful Laughter on Stress & Natural Killer Cell Cytotoxicity, January 1997 137.

Haig, RA. *The Anatomy of Humor: Biopsychosocial and Therapeutic Perspectives.* Thomas, 1988.

Kataria, M. *Laughter Yoga Information Booklet: Your Happiness Guide— All You Need to Know about Laughter Yoga.* htpa.wildapricot.org/resources/Documents/LaughterYoga-Info-Booklet.pdf. Accessed April 2017.

Laughter Therapy: Cancer Treatment Centers of America. cancercenter.com/treatments/laughter-therapy. Accessed April 2017

Mora-Ripoll, R. "Potential Health Benefits of Simulated Laughter: A Narrative Review of the Literature and Recommendations for Future Research." *Complementary Therapies in Medicine* 19, no. 3 (2011): 170-77. lachyoga-sonne.de/wp-content/uploads/2015/11/Potential-health-benefits-of-simulated-laughter.pdf.

Pasquali, E. "Learning to Laugh: Humor as Therapy." *Journal of Psychosocial Nursing and Mental Health Services* 28, no. 3 (1990): 31-42.

Seaward, BL. *Managing Stress: Principles and Strategies for Health and Well-Being.* 8th ed. Jones and Bartlett, 2015.

Strean, WB. "Laughter Prescription." *Canadian Family Physician* 55, no. 10 (2009): 965–967.

Shelley, C. "Plato on the Psychology of Humor." *Humor—International Journal of Humor Research* 16, no. 4 (2003): 351-367. doi: 10.1515/humr.2003.020

Snyder, M, Lindquist, R, &, Smith, K. "Humor." *Complementary/Alternative Therapies in Nursing.* 5th ed. Springer, 2006.

Tse, MMY, et al. "Humor Therapy: Relieving Chronic Pain and Enhancing Happiness for Older Adults." *Journal of Aging Research* (2010): 343574. PMC.

Walter, M, Hänni, B, Haug, M, Amrhein, I, Krebs-Roubicek, E, Müller-Spahn, F, & Savaskan, E. "Humour Therapy in Patients with Late-Life Depression or Alzheimer's Disease: A Pilot Study." *International Journal Of Geriatric Psychiatry* 22, no. 1 (2007): 77-83.

Weisenberg, M, Tepper, I, & Schwarzwald, J. "Humor as a Cognitive Technique for Increasing Pain Tolerance." *Pain* 63, no. 2 (1995): 207–212.

Wren, KR & Norred, CL. "Healing With the Mind-Humor Therapy." *Real World Nursing Survival Guide: Complementary and Alternative Therapies*. Saunders, 2003.

JUICING
Valerie Tookes

Juicing is the act of extracting the liquid from fruit or vegetables, thus removing the bulk of fiber. Juicing makes it easier for a person to obtain a larger concentration of nutrients than by eating fruits and vegetables in their solid state.

History
The use of fresh juice to maintain health and treat disease is not a recent fad; instead, juices and their health-giving benefits have been recognized by healers for thousands of years. The word *juice* is derived from the Latin word *jus*, and it's primarily defined as "the liquid part of a fruit or vegetable." In ancient Greece, a common tenet was "let juice be your medicine." The use of juices as medicine predates written history; juices were used in a variety of ancient cultures throughout the world. Hippocrates, the father of modern medicine, was a proponent of juices and other beverages for treating diseases and maintaining health. He referred to some juices, wines, and meads as "nectars of the gods."

Preparing fresh fruit and vegetable juices is one of the easiest and most efficient ways to take care of one's health. The juices provide a rich source of vitamins, minerals, and other important nutrients that the body can quickly put to use without using the energy necessary to digest solid food. The process of digestion requires time and energy, but fresh juices are virtually self-digesting, so the energy normally used for digestion is freed up for the body to use to repair and maintain itself.

Philosophy
During the process of juicing, the cell walls of the fruits and vegetables are ruptured, releasing an abundance of nutrients such as amino acids, vitamins, minerals, enzymes, and chlorophyll, which are then quickly absorbed by the body once the fresh juice is consumed. It is this abundance of nutrients that creates an energizing effect in the body. During the juicing process, the juice is separated from the pulp, leaving most of the nutrients in the juice without the bulk and weight of the pulp. For example, it would take about five pounds of carrots to make one quart of carrot juice. Eating five pounds of carrots daily would be a difficult, but drinking one quart of carrot juice is realistic. On average, the body requires two or more hours to properly digest fruits and vegetables when they are eaten in solid form. After digestion, then the nutrients are readily usable by the body. Juicing also makes it much easier to consume fruits and vegetables of many colors to ensure the widest possible array of nutrients each day.

Practices: What to Expect

A basic formula to making green juices, recently becoming very popular, is to start with a base of celery and cucumber. Add to that base one or two leafy greens, such as romaine, spinach, kale, collards, cabbage, or dandelion greens. Then add a choice of one or more of the following fruits: green apple, green pear, lemon, lime, or grapefruit, and other goodies such as broccoli stems, sprouts, ginger root, cayenne pepper, a wheatgrass shot, or E3Live. Another formula to keep in mind is to stick to a three-to-one ratio of veggies to fruit so that recipes can be nutrient-dense without a ton of fruit sugar.

The cost of juicing depends on the price of produce, but organic foods are recommended for further benefits. While juicing has many beneficial effects on your body, using fruits and vegetables laced with fungicides, herbicides, pesticides, and preserving agents can negate some of the beneficial effects. If organic produce is unavailable or prohibitively expensive, use a fruit/vegetable rinse before juicing. Non-organic apples and cucumbers should be peeled as it is very difficult to remove all pesticide residue from these foods.

Your body can only digest from eight to ten ounces of juice at one time, so for maximum benefit, drink one serving and wait one hour before consuming your next glass.

Best Suited for These Conditions

- Heart disease
- Certain cancers
- Alzheimer's disease
- Arthritis and other inflammatory conditions
- Most chronic degenerative diseases
- Weight loss or weight management
- Slowing down the aging process

Coaching Tip

Juicing is a direct way to get a lot of nutrients into the body at one time but a client may ask if they can buy commercial juices for the sake of convenience. A tip is to let them know that to get the full benefits they must keep it fresh. Commercial juices are heat-pasteurized so the products can sit on the supermarket shelf; this process kills the vital nutrients. You can also advise them that most of the produce that goes into their juice should be organic (when possible) to get the most nutrients and avoid pesticides. Organic produce can seem more expensive but some conventionally-grown fruits and veggies are perfectly fine to buy so in order to make sure their dollars are spent well, have them check out the list

of the Dirty Dozen and Clean Fifteen, which can be found
at: ewg.org/foodnews.

Contraindications

- Juice has a potential adverse reaction to prescription drugs
- Juice is low in protein and healthy fats
- Juice's lack of fiber may cause digestive issues
- Large amounts of vegetable-based juice may cause gas, bloating, and diarrhea
- Juices may affect the thyroid: cruciferous vegetables contain a compound that can interfere with iodine absorption, which is necessary for your body to make thyroid hormones
- Juice may cause light-headedness if you're not getting enough calories to sustain you
- Sweet fruits should be avoided if you have candidiasis
- Fruit sugar does not immediately require insulin for processing, but may pose a problem for some diabetics
- Processed "juice drinks" contain high levels of unhealthy corn syrup and other refined sugars

Research and Benefits

Quality of life begins with the quality of foods that sustain it—we are what we eat. The most direct path to health and energy begins with a diet rich in natural foods such as whole grains, legumes, fruits, and vegetables. Unfortunately, the standard American diet (SAD) does not provide adequate levels of fruits and vegetables even though the Surgeon General, the US Department of Health and Human Services, the National Cancer Institute, the American Heart Association (Murray), and many other experts agree that fresh fruits and vegetables are key to good nutrition.

Juicing is seen as an efficient way to increase the consumption of plant compounds in a concentrated form that is easily absorbed by the body. Extensive research has established the link between the SAD and the development of the primary "diseases of civilization," such as heart disease, cancer, stroke, high blood pressure, diabetes, gallstones, arthritis, and many more.

A vast number of substances (known as chemopreventers or phytochemicals) found in fruit and vegetables are known to lower cancer risk. These include carotenes, chlorophyll, flavonoids, dietary fiber, and enzymes that work in concert with nutritional antioxidants like vitamin C, vitamin E, and selenium. The most common dietary recommendation is to consume a "rainbow" diet, focusing on colorful fruits and vegetables which will provide the body with the full array of pigments with powerful antioxidant effects, as well as the nutrients it needs for optimal functioning and protection against disease. Juicing is an easy way to color your diet with these foods.

References

Bailey, S & Trivieri, L. *Juice Alive: The Ultimate Guide to Juicing Remedies*. Square One Publishers, Inc., 2007.

Bavington, J. "Juicing—Contraindications." *MyBestRemedies.com*. Midnight Illusions, 2009. Web. 10 Apr. 2017.

Calbom, C & Calbom, J. "Juicing, Fasting, and Detoxing for Life."

Carr, K. "Green Juicing: Delicious Juice Recipe, Video & FAQs." *KrisCarr.com*. N.p., 16 Jan. 2017. Accessed 10 Apr. 2017

Keane, M. *Juicing for Life*. Penguin, 1992.

Minger, D. "What Are the Dangers of Juicing?" livestrong.com. Leaf Group, 12 Mar. 2014. Accessed 10 Apr. 2017.

Murray, MT. *The Complete Book of Juicing, Revised and Updated: Your Delicious Guide to Youthful Vitality*. Clarkson Potter, 2013.

Nguyen, A. "Juicing for Health and Weight Loss." WebMD, 2012. Accessed 10 Apr. 2017.

MACROBIOTICS
Sakura Okamura

Macrobiotics is a philosophy and an approach to eating and to life that enhances natural harmony through finding a balance between the opposing forces of yin and yang.

History

Macrobiotics was developed by George Ohsawa (1893-1966) during the 1920s. He overcame severe tuberculosis when he was 18 years old by following a diet developed by the physician Sagen Ishizuka (1850-1910). It consisted of brown rice, vegetables, salt, and oil; the diet was promoted in Ishizuka's movement called *Shoku-Yo Kai*, "Food-Cure Society." (Kotzsch, 31)

The word *macrobiotic* (from the Greek *macro* meaning "great" and *bio* meaning "life") was coined by German physician Christoph von Hufeland in 1796. Ohsawa employed the word to spread his diet theory and lifestyle practice worldwide, in the pursuit of people's happiness and world peace (Brown, 8 and Kushi, 171). Ohsawa and his partner traveled to European countries in the 1930s. Ohsawa's students, such as Michio Kushi (1926-2014), spread macrobiotics across the US after World War II (Kushi, 169). Macrobiotics was associated with other Eastern philosophies and practices, such as Zen, which was also being introduced to the Western world. As more people recovered from their illnesses through the macrobiotic diet and lifestyle, macrobiotics gained popularity as an effective healthcare modality and was well known throughout the world by the 1990s (Kushi, 168-169; Brown, 9).

Philosophy

Macrobiotics aims to help people become healthy and happy through finding a balance between yin and yang, and through being in harmony with nature (Kushi & Blauer, 21). The basic principle of the philosophy is called The Order of the Universe:

1. All visible and invisible phenomena are manifestations of Oneness.
2. All visible and invisible phenomena are different from all others.
3. All visible and invisible phenomena are constantly changing.
4. All visible and invisible phenomena have a beginning and an end.
5. All visible and invisible phenomena have a front and a back.
6. The bigger the front, the bigger the back.
7. All antagonisms are complementary

(Ohsawa, 2011, 102)

This principle is followed by the twelve laws of change of the universe, which describe the dynamic relationship between yin and yang (Kushi, 7). It indicates that nothing is neutral and that nothing has only yin or only yang. Everything has both yin and yang, and either aspect accesses the other. If yin becomes extreme, it produces yang—and vice versa. Macrobiotics shows us how to live in harmony with this principle.

From a macrobiotic point of view, "health and happiness are the result of living in harmony with nature, while sickness is the imbalanced or extreme" (Kushi & Kushi, 1993, 342). Symptoms of sickness are the manifestation of the body's natural attempt to restore balance. New Macrobiotics (Kushi and Kushi, 1993, 343) sees the yin-yang balance in every aspect of life, including food, weather, and shapes (see Table 1). Diseases are categorized in three groups:

1) excessive yin and lack of yang
2) excessive yang and lack of yin
3) excessive yin and yang, or lack of yin and yang.

(Kushi & Kushi, 1993, 344. See the examples of classification in Table 2.)

Table 1. Characteristics of Yin and Yang (Based on Kushi, 9, and Ohsawa, 2011, 32.)

	Yin	**Yang**
Tendency	expansion	contraction
Function	diffusion, separation	fusion, gathering
Movement	inactive & slow	active and fast
Vibration	shorter wave, high frequency	longer wave, low frequency
Direction	ascending & vertical	descending and horizontal
Position	outward & peripheral	inward and central
Weight	light	heavy
Temperature	cold	hot

	Yin	**Yang**
Humidity	wet	dry
Density	thin	thick
Form	long	short
Shape	expansive & fragile	contractive & hard
Dimension	space	time
Taste	sweet, sour	salty, bitter
Vitamins	C	A, D, K
Foods	Grow in summer or in tropical weather	Grow in winter or in frigid weather

Practices: What to Expect

There are macrobiotic consultants training programs worldwide. Macrobiotic consultants assess your unique conditions through investigating your yin-yang balance, which is manifested in appearance, symptoms, and lifestyle (see the list of the practitioner training); macrobiotic consultants help find a way to restore balance in your life. As macrobiotic diet and lifestyle are simple and plain, you can incorporate key ideas of the modality into your daily life.

What to Eat

The "standard macrobiotic diet" (Kushi, 35) consists of 40 to 60 percent whole grains; 20 to 30 percent vegetables; 5 to 10 percent legumes and sea vegetables; 5 to 10 percent soups; and 5 percent occasional animal products and desserts (Kushi & Blauer, 35-37; Kushi & Jack, 972). It is recommended to use as much local, seasonal, organic, and less processed foods as possible.

Figure 1. Macrobiotic Food Pyramid (Kushi et al., 2001, 3058S)

How to Cook and Serve

In addition to the foods themselves, macrobiotics recommends that you use clean water, ideally your local spring water, and that you keep your kitchen clean. In order to embrace the change of the nature and enjoy your meals and life, macrobiotics recommends that you use diverse recipes and serve meals with various plates that enhance them.

How to Eat

Firstly, make or find a place to eat where you feel relaxed. Before and after you eat, take a short time to meditate or pray for the foods you eat and the person who nurtured, delivered, and cooked them. Eat foods with gratitude and chew well. It is recommended to chew about 50 times per bite and to leave the table before you become full. Both drinking too much water while eating and eating before sleep should be avoided because they may interfere with digestion.

Lifestyle

Macrobiotics puts an emphasis on having a lifestyle which is in harmony with nature. Being exposed daily to nature, putting some plants in your house, and bringing fresh air into your room are often suggested by practitioners. Furthermore, choosing relaxing and natural clothes and non-toxic cosmetics and detergents are favored.

Being active is another component of macrobiotic lifestyle. As most health experts advocate, macrobiotics encourages you to go to sleep early, to wake up with the sunrise, and to do regular exercise because inactivity can lead excessive yin.

Best Suited for These Conditions

- Cancers
- Diabetes
- Digestive disorders
- Eczema
- Cardiovascular diseases
- Reproductive system disorders

Coaching Tip

You may refer a client to a trained consultant if the client needs professional macrobiotic treatment. Let the client know that during the session with the macrobiotic consultant, they may discover their symptoms and/or environment are mostly manifestations of either excessive yin or yang. It is helpful for the consultant to explain about macrobiotic theory and support your client to rebalance health. While there is no national or international credentialing, individuals and organizations across the country offer their own macrobiotic trainings. The resources below will help you find a consultant who meets your client's conditions.

Table 2. Diseases, Yin & Yang (Based on Kushi, 115-21 Kushi & Kushi, 345)

Excessive Yin	Excessive Yang	Yin and Yang Combined
Asthma	Colon cancer	Bladder cancer
Breast cancer	Heart disease	Depression
Colitis	Heart attack	Insomnia
Diabetes	Heart failure	Irregular pulse
Epilepsy	High blood pressure	Kidney cancer
Esophageal cancer	Ovarian cancer	Liver cancer
Hay fever	Pancreatic cancer	Lower stomach
Hypersensitivity	Paranoia	cancer
Leukemia	Prostate cancer	Lung cancer
Peptic ulcer	Psychopathy	Obesity
Pulmonary heart disease	Rectal cancer	Pneumonia
Schizophrenia		Spleen cancer
Skin cancer		
Tooth decay		
Upper stomach cancer		

Contraindications

Practicing a vegan-style macrobiotic diet can lead to a vitamin B_{12} deficiency, which causes nervous system disorders and anemia; B_{12} is especially crucial for the development of children's nervous systems. B_{12} deficiency can be compensated by regular seaweed intake and occasional fish consumption (Brown, 33-34).

If you change your diet to a macrobiotic diet, you may experience headache, light-headedness, fatigue, and extreme emotions as the toxic compounds in the fat are released to your blood. If you are used to eating less fiber, you may have diarrhea while your digestive system adjusts to a whole-foods diet (Brown, 2006, 53). Therefore, it is recommended to make a gradual transition to the standard macrobiotic diet.

Research and Benefits

As a macrobiotic diet is high in fiber and low in fat, it is both therapeutic and preventative for a large variety of chronic conditions. Among them, the most researched chronic condition that has been healed and prevented through a macrobiotic diet is cancer. Almost all components in macrobiotic diet are associated with anti-cancer effects. Whole grains are rich in fiber, and they have positive effects on estrogen, glucose, insulin, and oxidative processes. The second dominant food in the diet, vegetables, is also cancer preventative; 250 to 400 grams of vegetables and fruits daily decreases the risk of cancer by 23 percent (Kushi et al., 2001, 3058S). Soybeans, which are often used in macrobiotic meals, are beneficial for hormone-related cancers such as prostate, endometrial, and breast cancers. This is because soybeans are rich in isoflavonoid compounds that have antioxidant and antiangiogenesis effects (Kushi et al., 2001, 3059S). Seaweeds are also distinctive foods in this modality; they have antitumor effects on women's reproductive systems and on the thyroid (Kushi et al., 3059S).

A high-fiber diet is also beneficial for diabetes and cardiovascular diseases. An experiment with diabetic patients was conducted at a macrobiotic organization in the United States, and the results showed high vitality, weight loss, and reduction or elimination of medications after participants followed a macrobiotic diet for only a week (Lerman, 624). Besides fiber from whole grains, the macrobiotic diet is significantly low in saturated fat, cholesterol, and trans-fatty acids. Lerman, 624).

Practitioner Training and Credentials
Macrobiotics America—macroamerica.com
John Kozinski—macrobiotic.com

Resources
George Ohsama Macrobiotic Foundation—ohsawamacrobiotics.com
East West Center for Macrobiotics—eastwestmacrobiotics.com

References
Brown, S. Modern-day Macrobiotics: Transform Your Diet and Your Mind, Body, and Spirit. North Atlantic Books, 2006.
Kotzsch, RE. *Macrobiotics Yesterday and Today*. Japan Publications, 1985.
Kushi, L, et al. "The Macrobiotic Diet in Cancer." *The Journal of Nutrition* 131, no. 11 (2001): 3056S-3064S.
Kushi, M. The Book of Macrobiotics: The Universal Way of Health and Happiness. Japan Publications, 1977.
Kushi, M & Jack, A. The Cancer Prevention Diet: The Macrobiotic Approach to Preventing and Relieving Cancer. Revised and Updated. St. Martin's Griffin, 2009.
Kushi, M & Kushi, A. *Macrobiotic Diet.* Edited by Alex Jack, revised and enlarged. Japan Publications, 1993.
Lerman, R. "The Macrobiotic Diet in Chronic Disease." *Nutrition in Clinical Practice* 25, no. 6m (2010): 621-626.
Ohsawa, G. *Zen Macrobiotics: The Art of Rejuvenation and Longevity*. Revised, edited, and annotated by Lou Oles. The Ohsawa Foundation, 1965.
Ohsawa, G. *Cancer and the Philosophy of the Far East*. 3rd ed. George Ohsawa Macrobiotic Foundation, 2011.

MASSAGE
Christine Leonard

There is more wisdom in your body than in your deepest philosophies.
—Friedrich Nietzsche

Massage is a hands-on technique with a wide range of modalities involving the rubbing and stretching of muscles and connective tissues to relieve tension, rehabilitate and induce relaxation.

History

The history of massage is complex and can be seen in European cave paintings dated around 15,000 BCE, where the depiction of healing touch is shown in extensive pictorial records. In China, as early as 3000 BCE, the work called the *Nei Ching* contained descriptions of healing touch procedures and their uses. Massage is also included in the ancient practice of Ayurveda, an Indian tradition of healing dating back to at least 1800 BCE. Modern Western medicine began to take shape during the 6th and 7th centuries, BCE, in Greece. Then around 400 BCE, Hippocrates of Cos, became the "father of Western medicine," with his emphasis on not causing harm to the individual.

Hippocrates strongly supported the belief that "the physician must be experienced in many things, but assuredly in rubbing" for strengthening and relaxing the muscles. Massage was adopted into many traditions of Roman medicine and made its way through the Middle Ages, the European Renaissance, and Age of Enlightenment.

In the modern era, the massage we have come to know as common practice in the United States today, began in the early 19th century. A Swedish psychologist, Pehr Henrik Ling, developed his own system of medical gymnastics and exercise known as the Swedish Movement Cure. What has come to be known as Swedish massage is a system of strokes that create a very relaxing experience. The Swedish Movement was introduced to the US in 1856 by the Taylor brothers who studied in Europe, and subsequently by others, including John Harvey Kellogg who published numerous articles and books on massage, popularizing massage in the United States.

Philosophy

Massage is instinctive and has been practiced for thousands of years in all regions of the globe. The root of the word massage can be traced to the Arabic *massa* meaning "he touched or felt," or even the Arabic word *masaha* meaning "to stroke, anoint, rub." The Portuguese *amassa* means to "knead" and leads to the French *masser* "to knead, treat with massage." Today massage can be applied therapeutically to treat injuries or chronic conditions as well as to induce relaxation. There are a wide variety of massage styles and modalities from around the globe. An individual may try various sorts of massage to decide what is best suited to their needs.

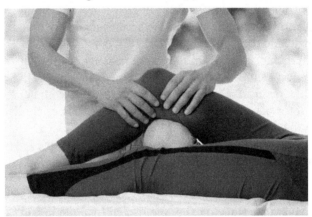

Massage Modalities

This list of modality and bodywork definitions has been collected from many sources for ready reference by the American Massage Therapy Association. (AMTA, Washington Chapter)

Acupressure: As a non-intrusive precursor of acupuncture, acupressure uses deep finger pressure applied at certain points located along an invisible system of energy channels within the body called meridians.

Amma Therapy: In Chinese, amma means "push-pull." Amma therapy is concerned with removing blockages and balancing the body's flow of energy along its meridians.

Aromatherapy: Aromatherapy is the use of essential oils for curative and rejuvenating effects.

Bioenergetic Analysis: Bioenergetic Analysis is a combination of physical and psychological techniques used to release constrictions in the energy flow of the body. Because psychological defenses are anchored in the body, special attention is given to the muscular patterns inhibiting self-expression. Developed from the work of Wilhelm Reich and refined by his protégé, Alexander Lowen, MD, this technique uses physical exercises, deep breathing, and massage to permit the body to give up its need to armor itself.

Chair Massage: When a ten- or twenty-minute relaxation session is needed, this is the technique for you. You are massaged fully clothed in a special chair designed to relax you.

Chi Nei Tsang: In Chinese "chi" means energy and "nei tsang" means internal organs. Chi Nei Tsang was originally developed by Chinese Taoist monks to strengthen their bodies to carry the energy required to perform their spiritual practices. Chi Nei Tsang practitioners work mainly on the abdomen with a deep, soft, and gentle touch to train internal organs to work more efficiently and to improve energy flow in the body.

Craniosacral Therapy: Within the craniosacral system is the cerebrospinal fluid that moves in a slight but perceptible tide-like manner. Craniosacral therapists assist in facilitating change in areas of restriction where this tide-like motion is limited, confined, and immobilized using gentle touch. Craniosacral therapy is helpful to those with nervous disorders, motor-coordination impairments, attention deficit disorders, insomnia, and other problems.

Deep Tissue Massage: Deep tissue massage is designed to relieve severe tension in the muscle and the connective tissue or fascia. This type of massage focuses on the muscles located below the surface of the top muscles.

Esalen Massage: Developed at the Esalen Institute in Big Sur, California. A very relaxing full body technique that is taught on a popular video published by the Esalen Institute.

Haelan Therapy: Haelen therapy recognizes that people who are in great pain are often unable to focus on the need to integrate body, mind, and spirit. It combines therapeutic touch, psychotherapy, and counseling.

Hakomi Therapy: Hakomi therapy is a system of body-centered psychotherapy that is based on the principles of mindfulness, nonviolence, and the unity of mind and body.

Holographic Technique: Holographic Repatterning, a six-step process of body/mind healing, acknowledges that our body's typical flight-or-fight response to stress creates non-coherent frequencies in our energy field

Hot Stone Massage: This technique uses stones that have been heated. These stones are positioned on the body and some are gently moved about with light pressure being exerted on the warm stones.

Infant Massage: Infant massage is usually taught to new mothers as a way of bonding with their newborn and of encouraging infant health. It incorporates nurturing touch, massage, and reflexology in a loving, fun, one-on-one interaction.

Integrative Massage: To assist in the release of emotional issues trapped in the body, long fluid strokes are used to move energy from the head down and out through the hands and feet. This is combined with the use of deep breath-work to aid the process.

Jin Shin Jitsu: Designed to heal the body by harmonizing its flow of energy, Jin Shin Jitsu a non-massage form of shiatsu, it uses 26 pressure points termed energy locks where fatigue, tension, or illness can trap energy.

Lomi lomi Massage: Hawaiian for "rub rub," Lomi lomi is a massage technique that's been handed down from ancient Hawaiian healers. Spiritual in nature, the strokes used are similar to the shiatsu technique of Japan but are gentler and shorter

Lymph System Massage: Lymphatic massage is very light massage, is very relaxing, and is used to promote healthy flow of lymph, the clear fluid that flows throughout our bodies.

Myofascial Release Therapy: Myofascial Release works by the manipulation of the fascia that connects and surrounds muscles.

Neuromuscular Therapy: Neuromuscular Therapy is a program of recovery from acute and chronic pain syndromes by utilizing specific massage therapy, including the pressure of trigger points, to eliminate the causes of pain patterns.

Polarity Therapy: By placing hands on various parts of the body, the practitioner connects the positive and negative poles to improve the flow of energy through the body and assist healing and relaxation.

Pregnancy Massage: This massage not only relieves the tensions and aches caused by the extra weight and shift in the center of gravity to the body, but it reduces swelling, soothes the nervous system, acts as a tonic, reduces fatigue, and enhances energy.

Rebalancing: Done in ten sessions, rebalancing utilizes a combination of deep tissue massage, joint tension release, verbal dialogue, and energy balancing to relieve physical pain, release emotional holding patterns, and enhance relaxation.

Reflexology: This is an acupressure type technique performed on the hands and feet and is based on the ancient Oriental theory that meridian lines or pathways carry energy throughout the body.

Reiki: Reiki in Japanese means "universal life energy." It is a healing technique of transmitting life energy by placing the hands gently in specific positions either on or above the body. This laying-on of hands is designed to relieve pain, restore vitality, heal illnesses, and aid spiritual growth

Rolfing: Also called structural integration, Rolfing was pioneered by American biochemist, Ida Rolf, PhD, in the 1930s. By manipulating the myofascial tissue in a ten-session series, each building on the previous one, Rolfers assist the body to reorganize, lengthen, and integrate itself into wholeness.

Rosen Method: This therapy, using gentle touch, breathing, and verbal interaction was developed by Marion Rosen, a physiotherapist, who noticed that clients who verbalized their sensations and emotions during treatment sessions improved more quickly than those who did not. The method applies gentle touch using hands that "listen" rather than manipulate. Rosen Method is used for both physical ailments and personal growth.

Shiatsu: Shiatsu, the most widely known form of acupressure, literally meaning "finger pressure" in Japanese, has been practiced for more than a thousand years in Japan. Shiatsu uses rhythmic pressure from three to ten seconds on specific points along the body's meridians by using the fingers, hands, elbows, knees, and sometimes feet to unblock and stimulate the flow of energy.

Sport Massage: This special form of massage is typically used before, during, and after athletic events to prepare the athlete for peak performance, to drain away fatigue, to relieve swelling, to reduce muscle tension, to promote flexibility and to prevent injuries. Depending on the needs of the athlete, a variety of techniques are used including classic Swedish strokes, cross-fiber friction, pressure-point work, and joint mobilization.

Swedish Massage: Swedish massage includes long gliding strokes, kneading, friction, tapping, and shaking motions.

Thai Massage: Thai massage is an interactive manipulation of the body using passive stretching and gentle pressure along energy lines. This ancient form of massage dates back to the time of Buddha and looks like a cross between shiatsu, acupressure, and yoga.

Trauma Touch Therapy: Trauma touch therapy is a ten-session certified program designed to meet the needs of clients with trauma and abuse histories. In a nurturing and unhurried manner, the therapist and client together create an emotionally safe environment in which healthy boundaries can develop, and respect and trust can unfold.

Tuina Medical Massage from China: Requires six years of university in China to become a practitioner. Works with the pulses of the energy pathways known as meridians in Chinese medicine.

Watsu: Watsu is a form of water therapy. Combining floating, cradling, stretching, shiatsu techniques, and dance-like movement, Watsu frees the spine, relaxes the muscles, and increases the flow of energy in the body.

Treatments: What to Expect

In a standard massage, there will usually be an initial intake form and confidentiality agreement. The therapist will also briefly interview the client to find a focus for the session. The massage table will be equipped with a face cradle and sheets in the case of a standard Swedish style massage. Many forms of massage require the client to be clothed and this will be articulated by the practitioner before the session. The practitioner may use massage lotion or oil along with various essential oils. The practitioner will use their hands, fingers, knuckles, forearms and elbows during the session with a variation of short, long, slow, and quick strokes. Quiet music is often an accompaniment to the dim lighting. At the close of a session the practitioner will leave the client alone to dress. There will often be an opportunity to discuss the session, ask questions and give follow-up recommendations.

Setting: Spa, chiropractic office, private massage therapy treatment office, or private residence.

Duration: 15–120 minutes.

Cost: $60–250 per hour.

Best Suited for These Conditions

- Anxiety (related conditions)
- Autoimmune disease
- Depression (related conditions)
- Fatigue
- Hypertension
- Insomnia
- Musculoskeletal conditions
- Pain—acute and chronic
- Pre- and post-partum
- PTSD
- Stress (related conditions)

Coaching Tip

Explore with your client their openness and understanding of therapeutic massage. They may have concerns about privacy, intimacy, professionalism, nudity, and vulnerability. Sadly, there is a lot of touch-adverse fear and negativity about safe and appropriate human contact in modern societies today. Discuss the various massage modalities, assuring them that something as simple as a heck-and-neck massage while sitting in a massage chair fully clothed might be a first step toward enjoying the profound benefits of massage.

Contraindications

- Not recommended on open wounds, sores, abrasions and burns
- Specific prenatal massage precautions are recommended during pregnancy
- Stored lactic acid and toxins in tissue may be released and lead to feeling ill or sore
- Certain massage modalities break up scar tissue or fascial adhesions and may lead to some temporary soreness and inflammation

Research and Benefits

Massage therapy has become one of the most popular types of complimentary/alternative medicine.

Pain management

Massage Therapy can help manage pain, both acute and chronic. Manual manipulation and relaxation resulting from massage can treat painful conditions, and has been shown to relieve acute pain in a postoperative setting (Adams). Massage can also relieve general muscle pain, back pain, and lower back pain (Ernst). Massage is also shown to help manage chronic pain caused by various conditions (Plews-Ogan) including headaches and migraines (Hernandez-Reif).

Stress reduction

Massage has been shown to elevate levels of serotonin and dopamine while decreasing cortisol, causing stress reduction and feelings of wellbeing (Field). Massage therapy can actually reduce symptoms associated with hypertension (Hernandez-Reif). Massage is helpful across the board for infants, children, and adults suffering from stress (Field). Massage benefits many conditions with associated stress symptoms, including pre- and post-partum conditions (Field), various stress disorders, PTSD, trauma (Rich), and even eating disorders (Hart).

Mood Elevation

Massage is beneficial for depression symptoms as well as treating chronic fatigue (Field). Massage can improve quality of sleep, reduce insomnia, and even give some relief during the end stages of cancer or renal failure (Cho).

Mobility

Massage therapy helps with joint rigidity and symptoms of fibromyalgia (Castro-Sanchez) as well as rheumatoid and osteoarthritis (Field). Massage can treat athletic injuries and helps with recuperation and range of motion post-surgery or injury recuperation and prevention (Weerapong).

Practitioner Training and Credentials

Massage training is organized by individual massage schools. Massage workshops are offered on specific modalities as well. In the United States the requirements to get a certification or license vary state to state and can be found on individual state board websites.

Some states require the national board exam and some have a specific state board exam, while still others have varying requirements individually, by city or county. Different states have individual requirements for number of educational hours in: anatomy and physiology, kinesiology, ethics, and various modalities as well as clinical practice hours. Continuing education seminars, trainings, and workshops can be attended in addition to massage school to complete CEUs or to broaden the scope and specialty of the practitioner. Requirements for certification or licensure vary from state-to-state and even county-to-county or city-to-city.

Resources

Associated Massage & Bodywork Professionals—abmp.com
American Massage Therapy Association—amtamassage.org
National Certification Board for Therapeutic Massage & Bodywork—
ncbtmb.org

References

Adams, R, White, B, & Beckett, C. "The effects of massage therapy on pain management in the acute care setting." *International Journal of Therapeutic Massage & Bodywork: Research, Education, & Practice,* 3 no. 1 (2010): 4-11.

American Massage Therapy Association (AMTA) amtamassage.org.

AMTA Washington Chapter: amta-wa.org/?page=massagemodalities

Castro-Sánchez, AM, et al. "Benefits of massage-myofascial release therapy on pain, anxiety, quality of sleep, depression, and quality of life in patients with fibromyalgia." *Evidence-Based Complementary and Alternative Medicine* 2011 (2010).

Cho, Y-C & Tsay, S-L. "The effect of acupressure with massage on fatigue and depression in patients with end-stage renal disease." *Journal of Nursing Research,* 12, no. 1 (2004): 51-54.

Ernst, E. "Massage therapy for low back pain: a systematic review." *Journal of pain and symptom management,* 17, no.1 (1999): 65-69

Field, T. "Massage therapy for infants and children." *Journal of Developmental &Behavioral Pediatrics,* 16, no.2 (1995): 105-111.

Field, TM., et al. "Massage therapy effects on depression and somatic symptoms in chronic fatigue syndrome." *Journal of Chronic Fatigue Syndrome* 3.3 (1997): 43-51.

Field, T, et al. "Juvenile rheumatoid arthritis: benefits from massage therapy." *Journal of pediatric Psychology,* 22, no.5 (1997): 607-617.

Field, T, et al. "Cortisol Decreases and Seratonin and Dopamine Increase Following Massage Therapy." *International Journal of Neuroscience,*115, no. 10 (15 Oct. 2005): 1397-1413. doi: 10.1080/002074505909564591

Field, T, et al. "Pregnancy massage reduces prematurity, low birthweight and postpartum depression." *Infant Behavior and Development,* 32, no. 4 (2009): 454-460.

Hart, S, et al. "Anorexia nervosa symptoms are reduced by massage therapy." *Eating Disorders,* 9, no. 4 (2001): 289-299.

Hernandez-Reif, M, et al. "Migraine headaches are reduced by massage therapy." *International Journal of Neuroscience,* 96, no.1-2 (1998): 1-11.

Hernandez-Reif, M, et al. "High blood pressure and associated symptoms were reduced by massage therapy." *Journal of bodywork and movement therapies,* 4, no.1 (2000): 31-38.

National Certification Board for Therapeutic Massage & Bodywork. ncbtmb.org

Plews-Ogan, M, et al. "Brief Report: A Pilot Study Evaluating Mindfulness-Based Stress Reduction and Massage for the Management of Chronic Pain." *Journal of general internal medicine,* 20, no.12 (2005): 1136-1138.

Rich, GJ. "Massage Therapy for PTSD, Trauma, and Anxiety." *Bulletin of Peoples' Friendship University of Russia. Series Psychology and Pedagogics* 3 (2013): 60-66.

Salvo, SG. *Massage therapy: Principles and practice.* Elsevier Health Sciences, 2015.

Weerapong, P, Hume, PA, & Kolt, GS. "The mechanisms of massage and effects on performance, muscle recovery and injury prevention." *Sports medicine,* 35, no.3 (2005): 235-256.

Mind Body Approaches

MINDFULNESS
Sarah DeVincenzi

Mindfulness is a term used to describe a variety of practices that can increase our ability to keep our focus and thoughts on the present moment. A formal training program for practitioners and coaches is known as Mindfulness Based Stress Reduction, or MBSR.

History
Although it is a relatively new practice in US culture, mindfulness has long existed in Buddhism as a form of meditation and has its roots in many other cultures as well.

Philosophy
By keeping our awareness focused on thoughts, feelings, sensations, and interactions as they occur in real time, we are able to be present for ourselves and others. By not allowing thoughts of our past experiences to define the present ones (good versus bad, right versus wrong, assignment of false meaning), we create the possibility for new perspectives, from which we learn and grow our connections to ourselves and others. Mindfulness is a skill used to improve health from the inside to out.

Practices: What to Expect
The beauty of mindfulness is that you only need yourself to do it and that it is available for free. For beginners a quiet place where you can sit undisturbed and practice mindful breathing, qi gong or another meditative practice is ideal. These formal practices are continued with the ultimate goal of remaining present and aware throughout your day as life unfolds. There are many formats for initially learning mindfulness at a varied cost:
Setting: Alone or with others, anywhere quiet.
Duration: A few minutes to an hour or more.
Cost: Free or low-cost apps.

Website
Palouse Mindfulness, eight-week self-paced standard MBSR, free—
  palousemindfulness.com/selfguidedMBSR.html

Apps
Headspace is free or upgrades for a fee—headspace.com.
Buddhify, $2.99 for 80 short meditations—buddhify.com.
Calm is free or upgrades for a fee—calm.com.
10% Happier: Mindfulness for Skeptics, costs $19.99 and includes
  personal coach—changecollective.com/10-percent-happier.

Books

Thich Nhat Hanh, *Peace is Every Step: The Path of Mindfulness in Everyday Life* (1992).
Mark Williams and Danny Penman, *Mindfulness* (2001).
Jon Kabat-Zinn, *Wherever You Go, There You Are* (2005).
Kelly McGonigal, *The Neuroscience of Change* (audiobook, 2012).

In Person Classes

These sites will help you to find a class or instructor near you; they also contain other great resources.

goamra.org/resources/find-program.

umassmed.edu/cfm/mindfulness-based-programs/mbsr-courses/find-an-mbsr-program.

contemplativemind.org.

Best Suited for These Conditions

- Physical health
- Cancer
- Chronic pain
- Diabetes
- Gastrointestinal disorders
- Heart Disease
- Inflammatory based conditions (most)
- Metabolic syndrome
- Obesity
- Sleep disorders
- Stress
- Mental health
- Anxiety
- Depression
- Eating disorders
- Obsessive compulsive disorder
- PTSD
- Relationship conflicts
- Substance abuse

Coaching Tip

If your coaching client expresses an interest in being more present in their daily life, reducing their stress level or opening up to an increased awareness of self and others, mindfulness might be for them. Given the recent popularity of mindfulness, it has become a bit of a "buzz word." When recommending it as a practice, be able to speak to the specific potential benefits individualized for each client. There is plenty of evidence-based research available on the outcomes of mindfulness practices.

Contraindications

There are no set contraindications for the practice of mindfulness, however caution is recommended specifically for clients with a history of trauma and psychological conditions. Some instances of increased emotional distress (anxiety, depression, panic) have been reported in this population when their attention or awareness becomes focused on a triggering topic. The suitability of mindfulness practice for each individual should be assessed on an ongoing basis

Research and Benefits

Practicing mindfulness, even for just a few weeks, can bring a variety of physical, psychological, and social benefits.

- Mindfulness is good for our bodies: A seminal study found that after just eight weeks of training, mindfulness meditation boosts our immune system's ability to fight off illness.
- Mindfulness is good for our minds: Several studies have found that mindfulness increases positive emotions while reducing negative emotions and stress. Indeed, at least one study suggests mindfulness may be as good as antidepressants in fighting depression and preventing relapse.
- Mindfulness changes our brains: Research has found that mindfulness increases density of gray matter in brain regions linked to learning, memory, emotion regulation, and empathy.
- Mindfulness helps us focus: Studies suggest that mindfulness helps us tune out distractions and improves our memory and attention skills.
- Mindfulness fosters compassion and altruism: Research suggests that mindfulness training makes us more likely to help someone in need and that it increases activity in the neural networks involved in understanding the suffering of others and regulating emotions. Evidence suggests that mindfulness might boost self-compassion as well.
- Mindfulness enhances relationships: Research suggests that mindfulness makes couples more satisfied with their relationship, makes each partner feel more optimistic and relaxed, and makes both partners feel more accepting of each other and closer to one another.

- Mindfulness helps veterans: Studies suggest that mindfulness can reduce the symptoms of post-traumatic stress disorder (PTSD) in the aftermath of war.
- Mindfulness fights obesity: Practicing "mindful eating" encourages healthier eating habits, helps people lose weight, and helps them savor the food they do eat.

Practitioner Training and Certification

There is not an established universally required curriculum to become a mindfulness teacher, however it is advised to seek out an instructor who is certified and well regarded in the mindfulness community. The American Mindfulness Research Association provides a list of formalized mindfulness research and/or training programs in North America and a few on other continents.

Resources

American Mindfulness Research Association—goamra.org/resources/find-program
The Greater Good Science Center—greatergood.berkeley.edu/topic/mindfulness/definition
Centre for Mindfulness Research and Practice—bangor.ac.uk/mindfulness
Mindful Schools for Educators—mindfulschools.org
Benefits of Mindfulness—helpguide.org/harvard/benefits-of-mindfulness.htm
Online Evidence-Based Behavioral Change Programs—emindful.com

References

Chopko, B & Schwartz, R. The relation between mindfulness and posttraumatic growth: A study of first responders to trauma-inducing incidents. *Journal of Mental Health Counseling*, 31, no. 4 (2009): 363–376.

Creswell, JD & Lindsay, EK. (2014). How does mindfulness training affect health? A mindfulness stress buffering account. *Current Directions in Psychological Science*, 23(6), 401–407.

Garland, EL, Farb, NA, Goldin, PR, & Fredrickson, BL Mindfulness broadens awareness and builds eudaimonic meaning: A process model of mindful positive emotion regulation. *Psychological Inquiry*, 26, no. 4 (2015): 293–314.

Grossman, P, Niemann, L, Schmidt, S, &Walach, H. Mindfulness-based stress reduction and health benefits: A meta-analysis. *Journal of Psychosomatic Research*, 57, no.1 (2004): 35–43.

Khoury, B, Lecomte, T, Fortin, G, Masse, M, Therien, P, Bouchard, V, & Hofmann, SG. Mindfulness-based therapy: A comprehensive meta-analysis. *Clinical Psychology Review*, 33, no. 6 (2013): 763–771.

Kabat-Zinn, J. *Wherever you go, there you are: Mindfulness meditation in everyday life*. Hyperion: 1994.

Ludwig, DS & Kabat-Zinn, J. Mindfulness in medicine. *JAMA*, 300. no. 11 (2008): 1350–1352.

Schoorl, M, Mil-Klinkenberg, LV, & Does, WVD. Mindfulness skills, anxiety sensitivity, and cognitive reactivity in patients with posttraumatic stress disorder. *Mindfulness*, 6, no. 5 (2015): 1004–1011.

MYOFASCIAL RELEASE
Michael Craigen

Myofascial release is a form of massage that stretches and releases the overly restrictive sheaths of connective tissue surrounding muscles and other structural components of the body.

History
The term myofascial refers to the sheath of connective tissue, known as the fascia, surrounding internal bodily structures, including muscles. There is no official origin of the term (Ward). The technique is built upon early work of Andrew Taylor Still, founder of osteopathy, and colleagues in the late 1800s. An osteopath named William Niedner, was likely the first to use myofascial release in the 1920s. Though he never wrote about or officially named the method, he employed a technique dubbed *fascial twist* that involved winding of soft tissues to release tension (Ward).

Janet Travell, MD, is said to be the first to use the term myofascial in medical literature in the 1940s. "Myofascial trigger point" began to be used more regularly in the decades following, appearing in peer-reviewed journals and gaining recognition as a factor in some pain syndromes. Travell started using the term *myofascial trigger points* in her published works beginning in 1976 (Ward).

The first exhibition of myofascial release as a technique happened in 1981 as the focal point of new soft tissue release classes offered at Michigan State University. In 1983, Travell and David Simons, MD, created the first manual regarding myofascial trigger points, entitled *Myofascial Pain and Dysfunction: The Trigger Point Manual* (Ward).

Myofascial release is now commonly incorporated in a variety of health and medical practices, including physical therapy, athletic training, massage, and chiropractic. Self-myofascial release can also be performed using the hands or tools, such as foam rollers, balls, and other smooth, rolling objects. Myofascial release shares common ground with other manual therapy techniques such as Rolfing.

Philosophy
The purpose of myofascial release is to treat soft tissues of the body to relieve tension (short resting length of spindles that prevents full contraction) or restriction (decreased electrical activity to contract muscles) that inhibits efficient use of muscles (Manheim). Fascia, which envelops most organs of the body, can become restricted or tense from various forms of trauma, both mental and physical (Spinaris), creating a palpable nodule and stiffening bands of muscle that causes pain (Travell).

Myofascial release applies a low load, long duration stretch to the fascia to alleviate symptoms by restoring optimal tissue length. (Ajmsha). According to Sam Kegerreis, professor of physical therapy at the University of Indianapolis, "It must be understood that myofascial therapy represents a philosophy of care rather than a series of techniques" (Kegerreis).

Osteopathy, myofascial release's parent discipline, promotes a belief in the body as an integrative unit with an inherent regulatory system that has the ability to heal itself, and that movement of bodily fluids and organs is vital in maintaining health (DiGiovanna). This applies directly to myofascial release, where the physical pressure applied by the practitioner or self will aid the body by allowing it to act as it should.

Practitioners are taught to respond to the sensations they feel through touch, and to constantly adjust the pressure on the muscle. The treatment is believed to affect the whole body's "greater fascial system" that connects all parts of the body (Manheim), "reflex relaxation" occurs when trigger points are addressed. It is advertised to be a more focused and potentially comfortable way of stretching.

Treatments: What to Expect

Prepare your clients that the first visit or two may be uncomfortable as the practitioners work to increase range of motion and loosen tight fascia surrounding the muscles, but the gains will be worth the initial discomfort.

Myofascial release practitioners are specially trained massage therapists, physical therapists, or chiropractors who work on massage tables. They often have additional pillows or equipment for positioning the body. Some use a technique called needling which helps to loosen and unlock frozen muscles

Setting: Professional office or client's home.

Duration: ~60 minutes.

Cost: ~$80/hour or $200–400 per month with weekly visits.

Best Suited for These Conditions

- Myofascial pain syndrome
- Venous insufficiency
- Back pain
- Neck pain
- Chronic pain
- Fibromyalgia
- Repetitive strain injuries
- Muscular imbalances
- Pelvic misalignment

Coaching Tip

As a quick and safe way to relieve muscular tension, myofascial release can easily be performed by most able-bodied individuals. Recommend to clients who complain of muscular tension in major muscle groups, and advise beginner clients to start off with light pressure and build up over time, especially if older. Recommend a physical therapist or personal trainer if in need of further instruction.

Contraindications

- Rheumatoid arthritis
- Aneurysms
- Tumors
- Diabetes (advanced)
- Osteoporosis
- Fractures

Research and Benefits

Research on the effectiveness of myofascial release is inconclusive. There have been many individual studies showing positive results. A 2016 narrative review showed improvements in range of motion through self-release techniques like foam rolling across numerous studies, but illuminated a lack of clinical trials, claiming a need for more to support the efficacy of self-myofascial release (Kalichman). A 2015 systematic review found self myofascial release to increase mobility and aid recovery acutely, but was inconclusive as to the long-term benefits (Beardsley). Another 2015 systematic review claimed the literature was mixed in both quality and results, specifically referring to inconsistencies in randomized control trials (Ajmsha). A 2013 systematic review acknowledged the existence of positive results, but again emphasized the need for stronger randomized control trials that are double blind, and that use practitioners who use the technique as part of regular practice (McKenny).

In a 2009 article by Robert F. Kidd, entitled "Why myofascial release will never be evidence-based," Kidd looks at myofascial release as an art form, and therefore tracking results to show effectiveness goes beyond results the patient experiences, but also needs to include the way the technique is applied.

Myofascial release has not been shown to have beneficial effects on cancer, though a 1996 study showed evidence of some symptomatic relief of chest wall pressure (Crawford).

Practitioner Training and Credentials

Currently, there is no official certification offered for myofascial release or self-myofascial release. The practices is often interwoven into physical therapy and chiropractic training programs. John F. Barnes, PT, a leader and major proponent of popularizing myofascial release, offers training seminars. Many other organizations and websites offer informal training through a multitude of media.

Resources
John F. Barnes' Myofascial Release—myofascialrelease.com
Becoming a Supple Leopard by Kelly Starrett
NASM Trainer on Foam Rolling: blog.nasm.org/training-benefits/foam-rolling-applying-the-technique-of-self-myofascial-release/

References
Ajmsha, MS, Noora R, Al-Mudahka, JA, & Al-Madzhar. "Effectiveness of Myofascial Release: Systematic Review of Randomized Controlled Trials." *Journal of Bodywork and Movement Therapies* 19, no. 1 (2015): 102-112, doi: 10.1016/j.jbmt.2014.06.001

Beardsley, C & Škarabot, J. "Effects of Self-Myofascial Release: A Systematic Review." *Journal of Bodywork and Movement Therapies* 19, no. 4 (2015): 747-58, doi: 10.1016/j.jbmt.2015.08.007

Crawford, JS, Simpson, J, & Crawford, P. "Myofascial Release Provides Symptomatic Relief from Chest Wall Tenderness Occasionally Seen Following Lumpectomy and Radiation in Breast Cancer Patients." *International Journal of Radiation Oncology, Biology, Physics* 34, no. 5 (1996): 1188-9.

DiGiovanna, EJ, Schiowitz, S, & Dowling, DJ. *An Osteopathic Approach to Diagnosis and Treatment.* 3rd ed. Lippincott Williams & Wilkins, 2005.

Kalichman, L & David, CB. "Effect of Self-Myofascial Release on Myofascial Pain,

Muscle Flexbility, and Strength: A Narrative Review." *Journal of Bodywork and Movement Therapies* (2016). Doi: 10.1016/j.jbmt.2016.11.006

Kegerries, S. "Myofascial Therapy." *The Myofascial Release Manual*, 4th ed. Ed. Carol J.

Manheim. Slack, Inc., 2008.

Kidd, RF. "Why Myofascial Release Will Never Be Evidence-Based." *International Musculoskeletal Medicine Journal* 31, no. 2 (2009): 55-56. rfkidd.com/myofascial-release-kidd.pdf.

Manheim, CJ. *The Myofascial Release Manual*, 4th ed. SLACK Inc., 2008.

McKenny, K, et al. "Myofascial Release as a Treatment for Orthopaedix Conditions: A Systematic Review." *Journal of Athletic Training* 48, no. 4 (2013): 522-527. doi: 10.4085/1062-6050-48.3.17.

Spinaris, T & DiGiovanna, EJ. "Myofascial (Soft Tissue) Techniques." *An Osteopathic Approach to Diagnosis and Treatment,* 3rd ed. Eds: Eileen J. DiGiovanna, Stanley Schiowitz, and Dennis J. Dowling. Lippincott Williams & Wilkins, 2005.

Travell, J, Simons, D, & Simons, L. *Myofascial Pain and Dysfunction: The Trigger Point Manual,* 2nd ed. Lippincott Williams & Wilkins, 1999.

Ward, RC. "Myofascial Release: A Brief History." *The Myofascial Release Manual*, 4th ed., Ed: Carol J. Manheim. Slack, Inc., 2008.

NATUROPATHIC MEDICINE
Meg Jordan

Naturopathic medicine is a distinct system of healthcare, based in the philosophy that the body has an inherent wisdom and tendency to self-heal. A naturopathic doctor (ND) supports the body's innate healing power through the application of natural therapeutics.

History
Naturopathy is viewed as a traditional form of practice that traces its history to Benedict Lust in the late 19th century. The European water cure and other Eurocentric practices of herbal therapy were foundational concepts. A decline in naturopathy practice (along with homeopathic and chiropractic) was the result of a federally sponsored campaign in the US and Canada to establish allopathic dominance in higher education, as supported up by the 1910 Flexner Report. But the popularization of holistic health movements in the 1970s generated renewed interest in the natural healing principles of naturopathy. Naturopathic medicine gained prominence due to the visionary work of John Bastyr, a pioneering educator who founded one of the leading naturopathic medical colleges, Bastyr University in Seattle, Washington in 1978.

Philosophy
The naturopathic medicine philosophy is captured by the Latin phrase *vis medicatrix naturae,* which means the healing power of nature. Traditionally, naturopathic doctors shared the perspective that the healing process is a matter of returning the whole person to health by reversing a disease process that often starts in the digestive system due to poor nutrition or assimilation problems. While that remains largely true, the NDs today embrace a wider perspective that includes genomics, epigenetic influences of pollutants, stress, mental states, clinical nutrition, traditional Chinese medicine, and acupuncture, as well as prevention and lifestyle counseling.

Treatments: What to Expect
A visit to an ND's clinical office may include a wide range of potential treatments including herbs and botanical remedies, specific nutritional and dietary advice such as anti-inflammatory or elimination diets, targeted vitamin supplementation, homeopathic remedies, hydrotherapy, acupuncture treatment, massage, advice about improving lifestyle choices, or an intravenous infusion of vitamin B_{12} or vitamin C. An invoice can be

generated for the patient who wishes to seek reimbursement from
insurance.
Setting: Professional office or clinic.
Duration: 60-90 minutes.
Cost: $100–400.

Best suited for these conditions

Naturopathic doctors often see people with complex chronic health
conditions that are not improved with pharmaceuticals or more invasive
procedures such as surgery. Collaborative research among ND researchers
and educators with MDs, osteopaths, chiropractors, and RNs has opened
new corridors of integrative care with evidence-based therapies. The
public's expanding awareness of the value and benefits of nature-based
medicines supports the growing demand for this approach.

- Naturopathic medicine is used to treat conditions like:
- Irritable bowel syndrome (IBS) and Crohn's disease
- Small intestine bacterial overgrowth (SIBO)
- Diabetes mellitus
- Metabolic syndrome
- Asthma and respiratory infections
- Eczema
- Fibromyalgia
- Seasonal affective disorder (SAD)
- Allergies and food sensitivities
- Chronic inflammatory conditions
- Chronic fatigue
- Thyroid problems
- High blood pressure
- Osteoporosis
- Premenstrual problems or perimenopausal conditions
- Migraines

Coaching Tip

Naturopathic medical doctors consider themselves patient educators as
well as experts in natural medicine. They offer their patients a generous
amount of time during initial visits to obtain extensive histories and teach
how to adopt healthier lifestyles. But as coaches know, being advised to do
something is not the same as doing it. Behavior change is difficult, and this
is where health coaches can offer their unique competencies to a
naturopathic medicine practice. Coaches can facilitate the needed behavior
change and mindset shift for the ND's patients. If you're a coach who
wants to work with NDs, tell them about the distinct advantages your skills

provide, and be sure to follow the specific clinical guidelines, learn about HIPAA compliance and align with their prescriptive advice for their patients.

Contraindications
There are no contraindications to naturopathic medicine practiced by licensed NDs who adhere to their scope of practice. If your client requires a drug, procedure, or surgery that is not allowed within the naturopathic doctor's state professional license act, then further inquiries can be made to licensed medical doctors, osteopathic physicians, or other appropriate healthcare providers.

Research and Benefits
The Naturopathic Physicians Research Institute (NPRI), a nonprofit organization, aims to increase naturopathic medicine research and analyses, and welcomes collaboration with interested parties. A growing body of scientific evidence supports natural therapeutics. There are too many findings to list in this guide, but for a more complete discussion of the numerous benefits and mounting research, read *The Clinician's Handbook of Natural Medicine*, 3rd edition, which accompanies the *Textbook of Natural Medicine*, 4th edition. These resources describe how natural therapeutics can be successfully used to treat over 75 of the most common diseases, along with therapeutic approaches for getting to the root cause of illness, rather than simply treating symptoms. The emphasis remains on treating the whole person and not the disease, while still knowing how to determine the need for conventional interventions.

Practitioner Training and Credentials
To earn the title, naturopathic doctor (ND), one must successfully complete a post-baccalaureate, four-year (or longer) accredited university or college of naturopathic medicine. Many NDs receive additional training in maternal care, earn midwifery certificates, acupuncture licenses, or become integrative oncology specialists. Depending on the state licensing act, naturopathic doctors perform physical examinations, take medical histories, order lab tests, and make diagnoses in their approach to treating illness and imbalances, just as medical doctors (MDs) do. In some states, NDs are licensed to incorporate some aspects of allopathic medicine into their practices, such as minor surgery with limited pharmacology and obstetrical examinations. With specialized training and additional certifications and/or licensure, they can also be midwives, homeopaths, and acupuncturists.

According to the Association of Accredited Naturopathic Medical Colleges, as of 2018, twenty states, five Canadian provinces, the District of

Columbia, and the US territories of Puerto Rico and the US Virgin Islands all have laws regulating naturopathic doctors. Proponents of formal naturopathic medicine education engage in state-by-state battles to gain recognition among regulatory medical agencies for licensure and legal practice statutes. Within integrative medicine, NDs are viewed as the leading experts in the art and science of natural healthcare.

Consumers should be aware of the distinction between NDs and the more traditional "old-time" naturopaths, who are not graduates of accredited naturopathic medical colleges.

Resources
American Association of Naturopathic Physicians—naturopathic.org
Integrative Healthcare Policy Consortium—ihpc.org
Academic of Integrative Health and Medicine—aihm.org

References
Hechtman, L. *Clinical Naturopathic Medicine.* Elsevier. 2018.
Murray, M & Pizzorno, JE. *Encyclopedia of Natural Medicine, 3rd Edition.* Elsevier. 2012.
Pizzorno, JE & Murray, M. *Textbook of Natural Medicine.* Elsevier. 2005.
Pizzorno, JE & Katzinger, J. *Clinical Pathophysiology: A Functional Perspective: A Systems Approach to Understanding and Reversing Disease Processes.* Mind. 2012.

NEUROFEEDBACK
Amy Flaherty

Neurofeedback, or EEG biofeedback, is a modality that empowers individuals to monitor and modify brain wave patterns for the purpose of improving health and wellbeing, and/or performance.

History

Observations of electrical current in the brain were first reported in 1875 by Dr. Richard Caton, a British physician and physiologist. Fifty years later, as German neurologist, Dr. Hans Berger, amplified brain electrical activity with radio equipment and recorded changes on graph paper and discovered that brain waves vary with changes in state of mind (Fuller).

Neurofeedback emerged in the 1960s when Joe Kamiya, PhD, and Barry Sterman, PhD, made profound discoveries relating to brain operant conditioning. Kamiya, a psychologist, demonstrated that participants could identify when they were producing a mental state associated with specific brain wave frequencies and that they were able to alter the amplitude when prompted to do so. Along similar lines, Sterman and his colleagues learned to train cats to increase their sensory motor rhythm (SMR) through reinforcement experimentation (Masterpasqua).

The work of Kamiya and Sterman precipitated interest in further studies relating to operant conditioning and the efficacy of brain activity. Since those early days, neurofeedback has become widely used to reduce the symptoms associated with many emotional, cognitive, behavioral, and physiological conditions, as well as to improve cognitive function and performance in healthy individuals.

Philosophy

The philosophy of biofeedback and neurofeedback (a subset of biofeedback) is a return of responsibility for one's own health. A self-control model, it differs from the traditional medical model in which a doctor may use medication, surgery, or other *external* controls to address an illness or condition. Through increased awareness and self-regulation of brain waves, biofeedback allows the individual to be an active participant in health maintenance (Fuller).

Brain waves occur at varied frequencies; different subjective experiences and mental states are associated with variant frequency bands. Ordinarily, individuals lack awareness of their neural activity and therefore are unable to influence brain wave patterns. Neurofeedback allows individuals to monitor their electrical activity on a brain–computer interface, promoting their ability to change their state of mind. Some frequencies are desirable and are encouraged; others should be reduced. With continued feedback, coaching, and practice, individuals are empowered to shift brain wave activity to a more regulated, desirable state.

Treatments: What to Expect

Because the training is specific to the distinctive brain wave patterns and symptoms of the individual, an initial assessment is conducted prior to commencement of neurofeedback. Some practitioners may do a limited assessment by placing one or two sensors on the scalp; others may conduct a more comprehensive evaluation, such as a quantitative electroencephalogram (QEEG) with the use of nineteen or more sensors (Hammond).

Once the assessment is complete and treatment goals have been established, one or more sensors are placed on the scalp and earlobes for neurofeedback treatment. The neuroelectric activity detected by the sensors is processed through software programs that provide audible and/or visual feedback via a game simulation on a monitor. The sessions are designed to encourage the individual to change and retrain their brain wave patterns through operant conditioning (Hammond).

Other practitioners have adopted methods of neurofeedback that work on different practice operating principles than traditional treatment, but often result in the same qualitative outcome. One such neurofeedback system is the Low Energy Neurofeedback System (LENS). This method uses weak electromagnetic pulses to assist in stimulating brain-wave activity and restoring brain physiology (Ochs). Another system of note is NeurOptimal®. This approach does not require an initial assessment or protocol created by a practitioner; rather, the neurofeedback system allows the brain to use its own input as a guide for self-correction. In light of this, NeurOptimal is considered to be brain training, not a medical treatment (Theoret).

Setting: Clinical office or home.
Duration: 20–25 minutes. 5–10 sessions or more.
Cost: $100–300.

Areas of Application

Neurofeedback has been found to be effective in the treatment of a variety of disorders and conditions. Research also backs the use of neurofeedback in healthy individuals for improvements in performance and cognitive abilities. Areas of application include (but are not limited to) the following:

- ADD/ADHD
- Peak performance training
- Cognitive and memory enhancement

- Alcohol and substance abuse
- Anxiety and depression
- Insomnia
- Concussions and head injuries

Coaching Tip

Encourage clients to keep a journal to note the changes they experience after or between sessions. This will help them to become aware of the shifts that occur as a result of the neurofeedback.

Contraindications

The majority of practitioners report that neurofeedback has minimal to no side effects; however, a few instances of adverse reactions have been cited. Mild side effects have included fatigue, agitation, irritability, headache, and sleep disturbance. In most cases, the effects diminish shortly after the training session.

Clients should make their practitioner aware of any adverse effects so that training protocols can be altered for future sessions (Myers).

Research and Benefits

ADHD/ADD

The most common application of neurofeedback is to Attention Deficit Hyperactivity Disorder (ADHD) and related disorders. Neurofeedback has been researched and applied to ADHD and similar conditions since the 1970s, and there is substantial evidence that demonstrates long-term effectiveness in increased attention span, improved retention and memory, stabilized mood, and reduction of impulsivity and hyperactive behaviors (Hammond). Among the numerous studies is one conducted by neuropsychologists, Dorothy Edgell and William Gaddes, who reported that 80 percent of children with ADHD who were treated with neurofeedback showed significant long-term improvements in IQ tests, standardized tests of achievement, and teacher/parent ratings of behavior (Fox).

Peak Performance Training

Neurofeedback training has proven to be beneficial for healthy individuals as well. Athletes, business professionals, medical professionals, and musicians/performers have used neurofeedback to enhance cognitive, emotional, and psychophysiological abilities (Pacheco). In many cases, the training is used to improve attention skills and insulate the mind from distractions. One impressive study involving microsurgeons-in-training deduced that after only eight sessions, participants demonstrated significant improvements in surgical skill and a 26 percent reduction in surgical task time (Hammond).

Cognitive and Memory Enhancement

Neurofeedback has been used to improve working memory and cognitive functioning in normal individuals, as well as to counter the effects of aging in those with cognitive impairment. There is research to demonstrate improved speed of information processing, resistance to interference, and enhanced neuroplasticity with the use of neurofeedback training. *The International Journal of Psychophysiology* highlighted a study showing a link between neurofeedback training and improved memory in a 40-person trial. Those who received neurofeedback increased their recall from 70.6 percent to 81.6 percent, while the control group showed a less significant increase (Imperial College of Science, Technology and Medicine).

Alcohol and Substance Abuse

Research supports the efficacy of neurofeedback as adjunct therapy for both sedative and stimulative drug abuse. The treatment allows an individual to better tolerate stress and anxiety, promoting a more calm, focused, and relaxed state. In a noteworthy study with 121 volunteers in an inpatient substance abuse program, 77 percent of subjects completing neurofeedback protocol were abstinent at twelve months, compared to 44 percent for the control group with no neurofeedback (Scott).

Anxiety and Depression

While these areas would benefit from further research, studies indicate that neurofeedback can be effective for treating anxiety and depression. Since anxiety often produces a state of over-arousal, and depression a state of under-arousal, neurofeedback training encourages self-healing, producing a more balanced brain, and resulting in a reduction of symptoms. One eight-week study involving neurofeedback treatment in patients with major depressive disorder resulted in reduced depression and anxiety symptoms as well as a decrease in clinical illness severity (Cheon).

Insomnia

Neurofeedback can be a powerful tool in helping to alleviate insomnia. The training works the areas of the brain that regulate sleep, improving the time required to fall asleep, sleep quality, and total sleep time. One controlled study demonstrated that only ten neurofeedback training sessions produced an increase in sleep cycles and a reduction of sleep latency (Hammond).

Concussions and Head Injuries

Neurofeedback has been used to address cognitive and emotional changes associated with concussions and head injuries. Treatment in traumatic brain injury (TBI) patients has resulted in improvements in learning, memory, and psychological wellbeing (Ataollahi). One study demonstrated that 80 percent of patients with mildly posttraumatic head injuries reported improvements in cognitive and neuropsychological symptoms after an average of 40 neurofeedback sessions (Reddy).

Practitioner Training and Credentials

Neurofeedback is practiced by a wide range of licensed or unlicensed healthcare professionals and may include psychiatrists, physicians, psychologists, social workers, registered nurses, educators, counselors, and coaches.

Providers of neurofeedback may choose to pursue a certification through the Biofeedback Certification International Alliance (BCIA). To take the written certification exam, applicants must have a BA/BS in a healthcare-related field from an accredited academic institution, as well as knowledge of human anatomy and physiology as demonstrated by completion of a human anatomy, human physiology, neuroanatomy, physiological psychology, or human biology course. In addition, applicants must have completed a 36-hour didactic education course from an approved training program, and have 25 documented hours of practical skills training with a BCIA-approved mentor (bcia.org).

While the certification is voluntary, practitioners must have the equivalent training and are required to follow standards and guidelines for the practice of neurofeedback that have been set forth by the Association of Applied Psychophysiology and Biofeedback (AAPB) and the International Society for Neurofeedback and Research (ISNR) (aapb.org).

Resources

Association of Applied Psychophysiology and Biofeedback (AAPB)—
aapb.org
The International Society for Neurofeedback and Research (ISNR)—
isnr.org
Biofeedback Certification International Alliance (BCIA)—bcia.org
The Biofeedback Institute of San Francisco—biofeedbacksf.com

References

Ataollahi Eshkoor, S, et al. "Mild Cognitive Impairment and Its Management in Older People." *Clinical Interventions In Aging* (2015): 687.
Cheon, E-J, et al. "The Efficacy of Neurofeedback in Patients with Major Depressive Disorder: An Open Labeled Prospective Study." *Applied*

Psychophysiology and Biofeedback 41, no. 1 (2015) 103-110. doi: 10.1007/s10484-015-9315-8.

Fox, DJ, et al. "Neurofeedback: An Alternative and Efficacious Treatment for Attention Deficit Hyperactivity Disorder." *Applied Psychophysiology and Biofeedback* 30, no. 4 (2005): 365-373. doi: 10.1007/s10484-005-8422-3.

Fuller, GD. *Biofeedback: Methods and Procedures in Clinical Practice.* 4th ed. Biofeedback Press, 1977.

Corydon, HD. "What Is Neurofeedback: An Update." *Journal of Neurotherapy* 15 (2011): 305-336.

Imperial College of Science, Technology and Medicine. "Researchers Find Link between Improved Memory and the Use of Neurofeedback." Science Daily, January 23, 2003. sciencedaily.com/releases/2003/01/030123073326.htm. Accessed April 2017.

Masterpasqua, F & Healey, K. "Neurofeedback in Psychological Practice." *Professional Psychology: Research And Practice* 34, no. 6 (2003): 652-656.

Myers, JE & Young, JS. "Brain Wave Biofeedback: Benefits of Integrating Neurofeedback in Counseling." *Journal of Counseling and Development* 90, no. 1 (2012): 20-28.

Ochs, L. "The Low Energy Neurofeedback System (LENS): Theory, Background, and Introduction." *Journal of Neurotherapy* 10, no. 2-3 (2006): 5-39.

"Overview of Clinical Entry-Level Neurofeedback Certification—Biofeedback Certification International Alliance." 2017. bcia.org/i4a/pages/index.cfm?pageid=3435. Accessed April 2017.

Pacheco, N. "Neurofeedback for Peak Performance Training." *Journal of Mental Health Counseling* 38, no. 2 (2016): 116-123.

Reddy, RP, et al. "Neurofeedback Training to Enhance Learning and Memory in Patient with Traumatic Brain Injury: A Single Case Study." *The Indian Journal of Neurotrauma* 6, no. 1 (2009): 87-90.

Scott, WC, et al. "Effects of an EEG Biofeedback Protocol on a Mixed Substance Abusing Population." *The American Journal of Drug and Alcohol Abuse* 31, no. 3 (2005): 455-469. doi: 10.1081/ada-200056807.

"Standards for Performing Biofeedback—Association for Applied Psychophysiology and Biofeeback". 2017. aapb.org/i4a/pages/index.cfm?pageid=3678#IV. Accessed April 2017.

Theoret, A. "Why Use NeurOptimal®? Neurofeedback for Anxiety." November 29, 2017. neuroptimal.com/learn/why-use-neuroptimal. Accessed April 2017.

PLANT-BASED DIETS
Valerie Tookes

A plant-based diet is a diet based on foods derived from plants, including vegetables, whole grains, legumes, and fruits, with few or no animal products.

History

A recent Gallup poll stated that five percent of Americans define themselves as vegetarian (Newport) and up to ten percent call themselves vegetarian-inclined (Vegetarian Times); the vegetarian segment of the population has remained relatively steady over the last twenty years (Newport).

The reasons for turning to a plant-based diet are wide ranging and include religious beliefs, cultural, philosophical and ecological factors, and health concerns. Ethical and spiritual concerns have motivated abstention from meat since ancient times, dating back to Greek philosophers. More recent philosophical reasons have been added in support of plant-based diets, including concern with how animals are raised in modern concentrated animal feeding operations (CAFOs), concern about killing of animals for meat, respect for animal rights, and feeling community with the natural world, including animals. These concerns are coupled with scientific arguments for the health benefits of a plant-based diet, a concern that first began to emerge in the 19th century and continues to be researched today.

Yet for all of its history, plant-based diets can be notoriously difficult to define in a uniform manner. The phrase *plant-based diet* has come to refer to a variety of diets that contain varying amount of animal products. It encompasses diets that include no meat at all (vegan) and those that include small amounts of any kind of meat with the primary focus of the diet being plant-based foods.

Philosophy

A plant-based diet can be used to refer to any of the following categories:

> **Veganism**: A diet of vegetables, legumes, fruit, grains, nuts, and seeds, but no food from animal sources. Within that category there are subcategories which include:
>
> o **Fruitarianism:** A vegan diet consisting primarily of fruit.
>
> o **Raw veganism:** A vegan diet in which food is uncooked and sometimes dehydrated.

Vegetarianism: A diet of vegetables, legumes, fruit, grains, nuts, and seeds that may include eggs and dairy, but no meat. Within that category there are subcategories, which include:

- o **Ovo-lacto vegetarianism:** A vegetarian diet that includes dairy and eggs.

- o **Ovo-vegetarianism:** A vegetarian diet that includes eggs, but no dairy.

- o **Lacto-vegetarianism:** A vegetarian diet that includes dairy, but no eggs.

Semi-vegetarianism or Flexitarian: A mostly vegetarian diet with occasional inclusion of meat and/or poultry. Within that category there are subcategories which include:

- o **Macrobiotic diet**: A semi-vegetarian diet that highlights whole grains, vegetables, beans, miso soup, sea vegetables, and traditionally or naturally processed foods, with or without seafood and other animal products.

- o **Pescatarian**: A semi-vegetarian diet with eggs, dairy, and seafood

- o **Pollovegetarian:** A semi-vegetarian diet with dairy, eggs, and poultry, but not fish or red meat.

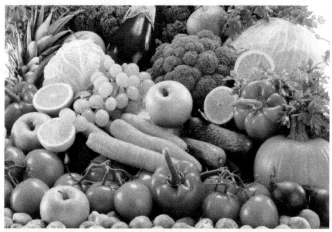

Practices: What to Expect

Practitioners should have a clear understanding of the differences between vegan and vegetarian diets, as well as knowledge of the various other subtypes of a plant-based lifestyle. When discussing these diets with clients, it is key to discuss the benefits as well as the potential risks of associated nutrient deficiencies. Since there are some potential risks and benefits with vegan or vegetarian diets, practitioners should discuss the reasons for their patient's diet preferences—weight loss, lack of availability, budget and financial pressures, or religious, spiritual, and ethical beliefs.

Practitioners may need to provide proper advice on nutrient supplements, fortified foods, and other strategies to prevent deficiencies. It is important to ask the client what foods will be excluded from their diet in order to assist in balanced meal planning and instruction on dietary supplementation. Clients need to be motivated to adhere to a plant-based diet, and it is the practitioner's role to point out that this will require planning, label reading, and discipline (Scuderi).

Best Suited for These Conditions

- Obesity
- Cardiovascular disease
- High cholesterol
- Diabetes
- Hypertension
- Some cancers

Coaching Tip

While health coaches should refrain from nutritional counseling or offering dietary advice, increasing your intake of fruits and vegetables is widely accepted as something most people need to do, according to the National Institutes of Health, the CDC and every credible agency that has surveyed the growing body of evidence. For clients wishing to improve their overall nutritional wellness, point out that credible experts recommend that a healthful plate of food is ½ plant foods (non-starchy vegetables and fruits), ⅓ whole grains and ¼ lean protein. Always recommend clients speak with their physicians, clinical nutritionists or registered dietitians for further dietary advice.

Contraindications

Potential deficiencies that can occur include:

- B12
- Protein
- N-3 fatty acids
- Zinc
- Iodine
- Calcium
- Iron

Research and Benefits

There is a growing body of evidence supporting the role of plant-based diets in reducing the risk of chronic diseases. As coaches, it is important that we encourage clients, whether they are vegetarian or non-vegetarian, to increase their fruit and vegetable intake and to limit the consumption of high-fat meats. The health benefits of vegetarianism far outweigh any risks associated with a plant-based diet. The biggest concern revolves around deficiencies of vitamin D, vitamin B_{12}, and iron; these deficiency risks are related to the severity of the restriction of the diet and can be avoided with meal planning and/or supplementation. If carefully planned, a plant-based diet can provide an adequate balance of amino acids, vitamins, and minerals, and the diet can provide sufficient calories to ensure good nutritional status (Sembrat).

Research has shown that there are myriad health benefits associated with the plant-based lifestyle. It is an effective strategy to reduce weight, to maintain a healthy weight, and to lower high cholesterol and high blood pressure (Scuderi). Vegetarian diets are high in fiber and low in saturated fat and cholesterol; further, according to White and Frank, vegans can consume between two and three times more fiber than omnivores. White and Frank's research goes on to show that there is a clear correlation between increased fiber intake and decreased incidence of colon, breast, and prostate cancer. Additionally, vegetarians are frequently closer to their ideal body weight throughout adulthood, which has positive ramifications in terms of decreased incidence of cancer, coronary heart disease, and cardiovascular disease (White).

Studies have also found that a vegetarian diet is associated with:

- lowered all-cause mortality;
- a decrease in risk of developing diabetes and improved insulin resistance;
- a reduction of hypertension and blood pressure;
- lowered risk for circulatory diseases (Scuderi).

Resources

Vegetarian Resource Group—vrg.org
Vegetarian Society—vegsoc.org
Academy of Nutrition and Dietetics—
    eatright.org/resource/food/nutrition/vegetarian-and-special-
    diets/vegetarianism-the-basic-facts
Physicians Committee for Responsible Medicine: Vegetarian and Vegan
    Diets—pcrm.org/health/diets

References

Berestiansky SL. "Vegetarianism at Each Stage of the Life Cycle." *Topics in Clinical Chiropractic* 3, no. 4 (1996): 14-24.

Clarys, P, et al. "Comparison of Nutritional Quality of the Vegan, Vegetarian, Semi-Vegetarian, Pesco-Vegetarian and Omnivorous Diet." *Nutrients* 6, no. 3 (2014): 1318-1332.

Daugherty, S. "Vegetarianism: Internet Resources." *Journal of Consumer Health on the Internet* 8, no. 4 (2004): 83-89.

Metz, M & Hoffmann, I. "Effects of Vegetarian Nutrition–A Nutrition Ecological Perspective." *Nutrients* 2, no. 5 (2010): 496-504.

Newport, F. "In US, 5% Consider Themselves Vegetarians." *Gallup Wellbeing* (2012).

Ruby, MB. "Vegetarianism. A Blossoming Field of Study." *Appetite* 58, no. 1 (2012): 141-150.

Scuderi, C, et al. "Is a Plant-Based Diet Right for Your Patient?" *Consultant* 54, no. 9 (2014): 1-10.

Tompkins, EK. "Plant-Based Diets." *Journal of Consumer Health on the Internet* 16, no. 2 (2012): 276-291.

Vegetarian Times. "Vegetarianism in America." 2008. Accessed on March 29, 2017.

White, R & Frank, E. "Health Effects and Prevalence of Vegetarianism." *Western Journal of Medicine* 160, no. 5 (1994): 465.

PLAY AND HOBBIES
Devin Hexner

Hobbies, or adult play, can be technically defined as a "pleasurable pursuit or interest outside one's daily work responsibilities through which one begins to make order out of chaos, e.g., botanical gardening" (Seaward, 353).

History
Why do we stop playing as we grow older? From the beginning of time, every animal instinctively engages in play—from the polar bears, to kittens, to monkeys, to humans—we all do it.

> *Play gives us the world, and through play we make the world ours.*
> —Miguel Sicart

Philosophy
Psychologists do not recommend avoiding stressful situations, however diversions like hobbies can be effective at reducing stress in healthy ways. There is a growing movement to spread awareness about the importance of adult play, through *hobbies*.

Hobbies can be activities like painting, making puzzles, playing basketball, cooking; simply put, a hobby can be anything we think of as enjoyable.

Hobbies can provide a healthy diversion, a mini-vacation, from the rigors of daily life like stress from work or family.

Giving your mind a break for some time can promote increased focus and attention when you return to more stressful obligations.

Additionally, hobbies can diversify your mental energy; if something at work or your social life becomes negative, there is a pleasurable activity waiting to alter your mood in a positive direction.

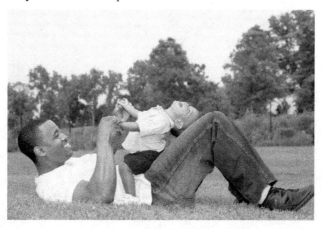

Practices

Active hobbies (e.g., playing music, making puzzles, painting, juggling), are considered especially healthy because they can boost your sense of identity and self-esteem; these hobbies often require creativity and project management. This can boost confidence and belief in your ability to manage other life problems.

Best Suited for These Conditions

- Chronic stress
- Anxiety
- Workaholism
- Depression
- Addiction

Coaching Tip

It is always essential for a coach to evaluate the right time to switch from the coaching role to a consulting role. When it comes to the topic of hobbies and adult play, this is an area where consulting a client can be especially effective for guiding clients to a greater state of wellbeing. Everyone will benefit from taking personal time to explore activities that break up the monotony of life. As a coach, it is useful to inquire with the client about what hobbies and activities have brought them enjoyment and fulfillment, and then encourage the client to carve out time in their schedules to play.

Contraindications

Everyone can benefit from play in the form of hobbies! Still, the saying "different strokes for different folks" is applicable, as one person's stress reliever might be another person's stress inducer.

Research and Benefits

Without play, life can become drudgery. Renowned researcher and psychiatrist, Stuart Brown, MD, has studied human behavior and animals in nature, and determined that engaging in play activities is critical for wellbeing and success in life.

According to Brown, when we stop playing, "You begin to see that the perseverance and joy in work is lessened and that life is more laborious" (Brown).

If perseverance and joy decrease, and life becomes more and more strenuous, stress must be increasing.

Dr. Brown founded the National Institute for Play (NIFP) for adults to increase their "Play Quotient," a concept created by Stevanne Auerbach, PhD. Known as Dr. Toy, Auerbach is a notable advocate for people of all ages to play. She has studied thousands of children at play over the years, and has shifted her attention to adults to increase their "Play Quotient." She asserts that as adults play more outside of busy work lives, they will be able to reduce stress, increase joy, connect with others, and stimulate the mind. More research is being devoted to play, and scientists have found "a significant reduction of anxiety level both in adult and aging rats" who engaged in play-like behavior with toys, as opposed to other rats.

Resources
National Institute For Play—nifplay.org/institute/about-us
TED Talk, "Play Is More Than Just Fun." 2008—
    Ted.com/talks/stuart_brown_says_play_is_more_than_fun_it_s_vital.

References
Auerbach, S. "Rx for Adult Play Year Round." *The Huffington Post*.
    TheHuffingtonPost.com. Accessed March 30, 2017.
Brown, S. "Play Is More Than Just Fun." TED Talk. 2008.
    ted.com/talks/stuart_brown_says_play_is_more_than_fun_it_s_vital
Darwish, M, Korányi, L, Nyakas, C, & Almeida, OF. "Exposure to a Novel
    Stimulus Reduces Anxiety Level in Adult and Aging Rats." *Physiology
    and Behavior* 72, no. 3 (2001): 403-07.
Greenberg, JS. *Comprehensive Stress Management*. McGraw-Hill, 2013.
Parks, AC. *The Wiley Blackwell Handbook of Positive Psychological
    Interventions*. Wiley Blackwell, 2014.
"Play Doesn't End with Childhood: Why Adults Need Recess Too." *All
    Things Considered*. National Public Radio. August 6, 2014.
Seaward, BL. *Managing Stress: Principles and Strategies for Health and
    Wellbeing*. Jones and Bartlett Publishers, 2015.
Sicart, M. *Playful Thinking Series: Play Matters*. MIT Press, 2014.

POLARITY THERAPY
Brooke Griffin

Polarity therapy is a comprehensive, holistic healthcare system comprised of a synthesis of therapies from ancient and modern health and wisdom traditions from the East and the West, including Ayurveda, Chinese medicine, homeopathy, chiropractic, and osteopathy. Polarity therapy was developed by Randolph Stone, DO, DC, ND.

History
Dr. Stone was formally trained and certified as a chiropractor, naturopath, and osteopath. He traveled all over the world, studying healing traditions and incorporating these lessons into his private practice in Chicago. "Polarity Therapy was developed over a period of 60 years of practice and study which began in 1912 and ended with [Dr. Stone's] retirement at age 83." (polaritytherapy.org/polarity-therapy/#history)

Dr. Stone moved to India when he retired and lived there until his death in 1981. The American Polarity Therapy Association (APTA) was formed in 1984 as the official professional polarity therapy organization, and it remains active to this day. Currently, polarity therapy is considered a gentle complementary energy healing modality and is often combined with craniosacral therapy, massage therapy, and Gestalt therapy or Somatic Experiencing.®

Philosophy
Polarity therapy is an eclectic, holistic, healthcare approach with a four-pillar system that includes body and energy work, verbal communication, energetic nutrition, and polarity exercises. In polarity therapy, there is an emphasis and focus on energy, which works on both the physical body and structure and on the energy field, and which is assessed and balanced through the lens of the Ayurvedic five elements and the Chinese concept of yin and yang. According to Dr. Stone, "Energy is the substance behind the appearance of matter and forms." (energyschool.com/about-cses/polarity-therapy)

Dr. Stone combined many healing arts and practices to effectively move blocked or stagnant energy in the system.

"Polarity Therapy is based on the premise that we are fields of pulsating life energy made up of specific frequencies known as the five elements: ether, air, fire, water, and earth. Each element relates and flows in a balance of positive and negative attractions arising from a neutral center. When our thoughts, emotions, and physical body are out of alignment with the energy necessary to meet a life challenge, an energy imbalance results.

These imbalances may appear as physical, mental, and emotional discomfort or pain. Polarity teaches us that this pain and discomfort is a signal for us to learn, change, and realign our lives" (Beaulieu, 2).

Dr. Stone talks about the direct approach to healing as being through life energy. "It is only the energy in matter that makes matter seem alive. When this energy escapes, only the shell is left.... A cure constitutes reaching the life current within and reestablishing the free flow of its energy." (Stone, 11)

Treatments: What to Expect

Polarity therapy works by balancing the positive and negative energy fields in the body, and by balancing the five elements of ether, air, fire, water, and earth. At times the practitioner will touch the body, and at other times the practitioner will work just above the body, not touching it. There are three different pressures and motions used, such as a deep, still pressure; a rocking motion; and a light touch. Clients are always fully clothed unless the session is combined with massage therapy. Craniosacral therapy is often incorporated into a polarity therapy session. Although a consultation on diet and polarity exercises is part of polarity therapy as it was originally designed, often this is not part of a modern day polarity session. Every polarity therapy practitioner will have a unique approach to the modality, and a unique emphasis or style. Polarity therapy is an effective healing modality for anyone who wants to experience benefits on all of the layers of the self, from the physical to the mental, emotional, and spiritual. It is an empowering form of healing that invokes one's power of breath and awareness, and brings balance to the whole being by allowing *prana*, or life energy, to flow freely.

Setting: Professional office with massage table or similar setting.
Duration: ~60 minutes.
Cost: $60–120.

Best Suited for These Conditions

- Emotional distress
- Physical pain of all types
- Chronic or acute conditions
- Digestive issues
- Constipation
- Sleep Disorders
- Stress
- Loss, grief, or bereavement
- Energetically out of balance
- Helping to let go of something

- Spiritual uneasiness
- Personal growth
- Muscle tension
- Depression

Coaching Tip

Each practitioner practices polarity therapy in a different way. Encourage your client to get personal referrals or read the biographies of various practitioners to determine with whom they feel a resonance. Feeling safe and comfortable with the polarity practitioner will enhance the effectiveness of the polarity therapy session. While many polarity therapists are also trained in massage therapy, it is more complementary if they are trained in craniosacral therapy.

Contraindications

- Cancer
- Blood clots
- Pregnancy

Research and Benefits

Although polarity therapy has been around for a while, and many who have experienced it and those who work as practitioners can attest to its benefits, there is very little scientific research available. Most of what can be found is anecdotal and personal first-hand experience. Polarity therapy is highly valued by many healing practitioners as an especially useful modality in trauma care. Although it is comprehensive on its own, polarity therapy combines nicely with many other healing modalities. The American Polarity Therapy Association has a section for the latest research available to its members (polaritytherapy.org).

Practitioner Training and Credentials

Polarity therapy training is approved by the American Polarity Therapy Association. There are three levels of training and certification. These are controlled by the Certification Governing Council of the American Polarity Therapy Association. The beginning training level is the Associate Polarity Practitioner (APP) with 155 hours of training. After completing the APP program, practitioners may complete the advanced training level, Registered Polarity Practitioner (RPP), which requires an additional 520 hours of training. After these two levels are completed with success, one can complete a total of 800 hours of training to be eligible to sit for the board exam. Passing this allows one to become a Board Certified Polarity Practitioner (BCPP). Recertification and continuing education hours are required every two years (polaritytherapy.org/certification).

Resources
American Polarity Therapy Association (APTA)—polaritytherapy.org.
Colorado School of Energy Studies—energyschool.com/about-
    cses/polarity-therapy.
Published writings of Dr. Stone—digitaldrstone.com.

References
Beaulieu, J. *Polarity Therapy Workbook*. BioSonic Enterprises, 1994.
Colorado School of Energy Studies. "Polarity Therapy."
    energyschool.com/about-cses/polarity-therapy.
Stone, R. *Health Building: The Conscious Art of Living Well*. CRCS
Wellness Books, 1985.

QIGONG
Kevonya Elzia

Qigong (pronounced chee gung) dates to before 200 BCE in China and is considered a component of traditional Chinese medicine (shen-nong.com). It is an energy medicine practice "for health maintenance, healing, and increasing vitality" that involves "a series of exercises/practices using posture, movement sequences, breathing patterns, meditation, and the mind." (Gascoigne)

History and Philosophy
Qigong means cultivating energy through the consistent practice of various specialized disciplines ranging from tai chi to kung fu. There are five traditions of qigong theory: Taoist, Buddhist, Confucian, medical, and martial arts. The traditions have similarities, however, the focus or intent of practice for each is different and falls into one of the following categories: martial arts, medical, intellectual, or spiritual. What makes qigong different from other exercise regimens is its utilization of the meridian channel system which is rooted in traditional Chinese medicine (TCM): mindful intent, breathing techniques, and rhythmic movement techniques intended to "reduce stress, increase vitality, and enhance the immune system" (nqa.org).

Treatments: What to Expect
When attending a qigong class, participants should wear loose comfortable clothing and comfortable shoes.
Setting: Classrooms, inside, or outside in a natural setting.
Duration: 60–90 minutes.
Cost: $0–25 or more per class.

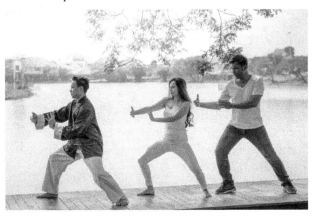

Best Suited for These Conditions

- Stress reduction
- Diabetes
- Improved balance/hand strength/flexibility
- Improved sleep quality
- Cardiovascular health
- Pulmonary function
- Fibromyalgia

Coaching Tip

Clients who wish to start qigong should look for a local community class and talk to the qigong instructor about their interests, physical challenges and desired goals. Encourage clients to develop a practice with consistency and learn to look for subtle changes in energy and equanimity.

Contraindications

- History of psychotic disorder
- Metal implants in key areas/points of movement
- History of an organ transplant

Research and Benefits

Research has shown that qigong has been beneficial for the following conditions:

Diabetes

Sun GC, et al. "The Effects of Qigong on Glucose Control in Type 2 Diabetes: A Randomized Controlled Pilot Study." *Diabetes Care*, 2010.33(1):e8. PMID: 20040671.

General Wellbeing

Zheng, Guohua, et al. "Qualitative Evaluation of Baduanjin (Traditional Chinese Qigong) on Health Promotion Among an Elderly Community Population at Risk for Ischemic Stroke." *Evidence-Based Complementary and Alternative Medicine* (September 21, 2015): 1-10. doi: 10.1155/2015/893215.

Cardiovascular Health

Zou, Liye, et al. "A Systematic Review and Meta-Analysis Baduanjin Qigong for Health Benefits: Randomized Controlled Trials." *Evidence-Based Complementary and Alternative Medicine* (March 7, 2017): 1-17.doi: 10.1155/2017/4548706.

Physical Rehab
Liu, Xiao Lei, et al. "Effects of Health Qigong Exercises on Relieving Symptoms of Parkinson's Disease." *Evidence-Based Complementary and Alternative Medicine* 2016 (November 7, 2016). 1-11. doi: 10.1155/2016/5935782.

Respiratory Health
Min, Zhang, et al. "Qigong Yi Jinjing Promotes Pulmonary Function, Physical Activity, Quality of Life and Emotion Regulation Self-Efficacy in Patients with Chronic Obstructive Pulmonary Disease: A Pilot Study." *Journal of Alternative and Complementary Medicine* 22, no. 10 (October 2016): 810-817. doi: 10.1089/acm.2015.0224.

Mental Health
Li, Jie, et al. "From Body to Mind and Spirit: Qigong Exercise for Bereaved Persons with Chronic Fatigue Syndrome-Like Illness." *Evidence-Based Complementary & Alternative Medicine* (October 4, 2015): 1-7. doi: 10.1155/2015/631410.

Fibromyalgia
Sawynok, Jana, et al. "Extension Trial of Qigong for Fibromyalgia: A Quantitative and Qualitative Study." *Evidence-Based Complementary & Alternative Medicine* (January 2013): 1-12. doi: 10.1155/2013/726062.

Practitioner Training and Credential
Depending on the type of Qigong and desired level of certification, basic credentials should include:

- 150-200 hours of formal training that includes clinical practice (not including books or DVD).
- At least two years of personal practice.
- Basic knowledge of Chinese Medicine theory.

Resources
National Qigong Association—nqa.org.
Institute of Qigong and Integrative Medicine—iqim.org
Acupuncture & Integrative Medicine College—aimc.edu.
Institute of Traditional Medicine—itmonline.org
The Journal of Traditional Eastern Health and Fitness—qi-journal.com
Oriental Medicine Journal—omjournal.com
Evidence Based Complementary and Alternative Medicine Journal—hindawi.com/journals/ecam.

References

Gascoigne, S. *The Chinese Way to Health: A Self-Help Guide to Traditional Chinese Medicine*. Charles E. Tuttle Company, 1997.
Institute of Qigong and Integrative Medicine—iqim.org.
Institute of Traditional Medicine—itmonline.org.
National Qigong Association—nqa.org.
Shen-Nong—shen-nong.com.

Subtle Energy Medicine

REIKI
Meckell Milburn

Reiki is a Japanese rest and relaxation technique in which Reiki practitioners channel universal life energy through their hands to help heal a client. Reiki can also be self-administered by practitioners to heal themselves.

History
Reiki as we know it today was discovered in the 1890s by Mikao Usui, a doctor of theology who was also well versed in medicine and philosophy. Usui, after years of academic study, embarked upon a quest to discover the concept of healing miracles through the lens of the Buddha and Jesus. Usui's curiosity was piqued by his own battle with illness, and he travelled around the world to find an answer to his quest.

After many years, Usui returned to Japan and discovered ancient tantric manuscripts that described a secret for healing the mind and body. Usui decided to travel up Mount Kurama, a mountain in Kyoto, for a 21-day practice of prayer and fasting in order to meditate on the information he had discovered. On the last day of the 21-day practice, after a powerful spiritual experience, he ran to tell his colleagues about it, and stubbed his toe, tripping on the exposed roots of the cedar trees that cover Mount Kurama. Like most people who have been injured, his reflex prompted him to immediately grab his foot; but instead of simply feeling the pressure of his own grip, Usui felt healing energy flow through his hands. Because this energy flow healed Usui's injury, he was prompted to teach many others this method, now known worldwide as Reiki. In 1922, Usui opened his first Reiki school in Harajuku, Tokyo.

It is important to note that although popularized by Usui, Reiki was not *invented* by Usui, but was *rediscovered*. Because the texts had been in existence for several thousand years, it is understood that others before Usui had engaged in similar practices, such as palm healing. However, Usui did help to frame Reiki as we know it today.

Philosophy
The word, Reiki, is comprised of the Japanese words *Rei* and *Ki*, meaning, respectively, "universal life" and "energy." It is believed that the Reiki force can be found flowing through all beings. Reiki energy, however, needs unobstructed channels in order to flow effectively. Physical, mental, spiritual, and emotional maladies are believed to be caused by energy blockages. Through Reiki sessions, practitioners aim to provide clients with an avenue to heal by unblocking their energy channels and allowing

the return of a natural flow of energy throughout the body. Regular Reiki sessions, whether practitioners are performing Reiki on themselves or on other people, are thought to accelerate the healing process. While healing others, practitioners are being healed themselves by the Reiki energy flowing through them.

Reiki practitioners believe that this Japanese healing modality spans religions and can be accessed by people from different backgrounds and experiences. Reiki's healing energy surrounds all. Reiki can be used as a primary modality or as a complement to other healing or medical interventions.

Usui Shiki Ryoho (literally translated to "Usui-style treatment") was the first style of Reiki, created by Mikao Usui himself. Usui Shiki Ryoho operates on four main principles: healing practice (healing via the laying of the hands), personal development (understanding that this practice creates daily life choices that can move practitioners closer to their authenticity), spiritual discipline (seeing Reiki as a spiritual path for practitioners), and mystic order (using Reiki to bring a sense of connection and purpose with others on this path). There have since been many other styles of Reiki created, including Karuna, Tibetan, and Kundalini. Each style of Reiki has a slightly different guiding philosophy, yet all are rooted in Usui Shiki Ryoho.

Treatments: What to Expect

Before a treatment, practitioners will often talk to clients about what they can expect, any specific reasons they are seeking Reiki, or any particular areas they would like to focus on.

Clients are fully clothed and in a comfortable position on a massage table or in a chair. Sessions typically take place in a quiet environment, but may take place in community settings and at events.

During treatments, Reiki energy is channeled through the practitioner's hands to provide healing to the self or others. Practitioners may provide treatments with their hands either directly in contact with the client's body, or hovering slightly above the client's body, or long-distance/remotely, with no direct contact with the body at all.

Full treatments involve practitioners channeling Reiki to various parts of the body for two to five minutes for hand position. Positions usually cover most of the front, back, and head of the body, targeting major organ systems as well as physical, mental, emotional, and spiritual energies.

During a session, clients may feel tingling, warmth, or no sensation at all. Areas that people feel more sensation in are said to be "taking more Reiki." Taking more Reiki may mean that the client needed more healing in particular areas, but it does not imply that something is necessarily wrong with that area of the client's body.

Reiki can be done on the self and can be practiced regularly as self-care.
Setting: Quiet setting with massage table or a comfortable chair.
Duration: 60-90 minutes.
Cost: $60–120.

Best Suited for These Conditions

- Anxiety
- Chronic pain
- Cognition issues related to dementia/Alzheimer's
- Depression
- Emotional pain
- Hypertension
- Increased heart rate
- Musculoskeletal disorders
- Preoperative stress
- Postoperative pain
- Stress

Coaching Tip

Reiki may be recommended for clients who are experiencing spiritual or emotional blockages, stress, or pain. Clients should seek Reiki practitioners who have been certified by a reputable Reiki Master, a practitioner with whom they feel comfortable. It is appropriate for clients to ask questions if they are unsure about the process or need additional information about what to expect during a session. Coaches can utilize wisdom that clients may have gained from a Reiki session to support their work in the coaching relationship.

Contraindications

Reiki is safe for most people, but must be performed only on those who have consented. Reiki may not be recommended for an individual who is experiencing unmanaged psychosis or someone who is in a coma.

Research and Benefits

There has been ample research in the last ten years or more on the benefits of Reiki. Institutions like the National Institutes of Health's National Center for Complementary and Integrative Health, as well as the Center for Reiki Research, have collected data on the positive effects of this technique.

In one study on stress published in the *Journal of Integrative Medicine*, college students taught self-Reiki were able to significantly reduce their stress throughout finals and saw continued effects twenty-weeks post-study (Bukowski, 336). Similarly, results of Reiki therapy performed on clinicians in a community mental health clinic showed a marked reduction in burnout compared to groups that received "sham Reiki" (Reiki performed by non-practitioners) (Rosada, 489).

Research on using Reiki for pain reduction is growing. One study on women who had just had cesarean sections found that a Reiki treatment after incision helped to reduce pain by more than 75 percent. (Midilli, 368)

Due to the increase of scientific evidence on the effects of Reiki in recent years, the quantity of research is expected to continue growing.

Practitioner Training and Credentials

There are three levels of Reiki practitioners: Level I, Level II, and Reiki Master.

To become a Reiki I practitioner, one must only decide consciously that this is the right time to become certified. Reiki I trainings must be done by a certified Reiki Master; they involve the Reiki Master conducting *attunements* to the students. During this process, students receive symbols, or words in Japanese kanji, that help to improve the flow of life force energy. Attunements connect students to the Reiki source through opening the crown and heart chakras, as well as creating a link to the source through one's palms. Once certified as a Reiki I practitioner, students are able to provide Reiki on a physical level to people, plants, and animals. The cost of a Reiki I training session ranges from $150 to $300.

To become a Reiki II practitioner, students must have completed Reiki I training and must have practiced Reiki for at least several months. Attunements during the Reiki II training increase access to the Reiki energy, and additional symbols are transmitted during this time. Reiki II practitioners may provide Reiki on mental and emotional levels in addition to physical levels. Reiki II practitioners can also perform Reiki long-distance, with consent, for clients. Reiki II trainings average $500.

Reiki Masters teach Reiki I and Reiki II, and they offer attunements to initiate students as Reiki practitioners. Reiki Masters have received, through attunements, the master symbol, which further increases the Reiki energy flow. Certification varies depending upon the teacher. All Masters must have taken Reiki I and II. Some teachers require an internship and a set number of hours providing Reiki. People are not full Reiki Masters until they teach Reiki to another person and pass on the symbols.

Once attuned, practitioners are forever able to access the Reiki energy and do not need follow-up attunements. However, the more practitioners work with the Reiki energy, the stronger the connection grows.

Currently, there is no regulation for practitioners in the United States.

Resources
National Center for Complementary and Integrative Health—
   nccih.nih.gov/health/reiki
International Center for Reiki Training—Reiki.org
The Center for Reiki Research—centerforReikiresearch.org
International Association of Reiki Professionals—iarp.org
The Original Reiki Handbook of Dr. Mikao Usui by Mikao Usui &
   Christine Grimm

References
Baldwin, AL, et al. "Reiki Improves Heart Rate Homeostasis in Laboratory Rats." *The Journal of Alternative and Complementary Medicine* 14, no. 4 (2008): 417-422.

Baldwin, A. "Reiki, The Scientific Evidence." *Reiki News Magazine* Fall 2011: 29-31.

Bier, D. "Reiki Healing and Mental Health: What the Research Shows." psychcentral.com/lib/reiki-healing-and-mental-health-what-the-research-shows. Accessed March 21, 2017.

Birocco, N, et al. "The Effects of Reiki Therapy on Pain and Anxiety in Patients Attending a Day Oncology and Infusion Services Unit." *The American Journal of Hospice and Palliative Medicine* 9, no. 4 (2012): 290-294. doi: 10.1177/1049909111420859.

Bukowski, EL. "The Use of Self-Reiki for Stress Reduction and Relaxation." *Journal of Integrative Medicine* 13, no. 5 (2015): 336-340.

Crawford, S, et al. "Using Reiki to Decrease Memory and Behavior Problems in Mild Cognitive Impairment and Mild Alzheimer's Disease." *The Journal of Alternative and Complementary Medicine* 12, no. 9 (2006): 911-913.

Kurebayashi, L, et al. "Massage and Reiki Used to Reduce Stress and Anxiety: Randomized Clinical Trial." *Latin American Journal of Nursing* 24, no. 2834 (2016).

Midilli, T & Gunduzoglu, N. "Body after Cesarean Section Surgery A Single-Blinded, Randomized, Double-Controlled Study." *Holistic Nursing Practice* 30, no. 6 (2016): 368-378.

Rosada, R. "Reiki Reduces Burnout among Community Mental Health Clinicians." *The Journal of Alternative and Complementary Medicine* 21, no. 8 (2015): 489-495.

Vitale, A. "An Integrative Review of Reiki Touch Therapy Research." *Holistic Nursing Practice* 21, no. 4 (2007): 167-179.

SHAMANISM
Meg Jordan

Considered the earliest healing tradition in the world, shamanism is an ancient practice whereby the shaman engages with non-ordinary states of consciousness and spiritual realms for the sake of spiritual growth, healing, or divination for self, another or a community.

History

The word *shaman* has its origins in the oldest languages of Siberia and Central Asia, where some of the earliest archaeological records (cave art) are 25,000 years old, and ritual artifacts (drums, masks, clothing) of shamanism among nomadic or herding cultures date back to the 12th century CE (Ekrem). The spread of dominant religious through colonization suppressed the common feature of accessing spiritual resources throughout much of the world.

Core shamanism is a term coined by Michael and Sandra Harner at the Foundation for Shamanic Studies to describe more universal, cross-cultural features of shamanism. With training in core techniques such repetitive drumming or sonic driving (rattle shaking to achieve trance states), the Harners believe that individuals can restore a rightful spiritual heritage. They also emphasize that specific ceremonies or sacred rituals of Native American or other medicine men and women should never be co-opted.

Philosophy

The shamanic worldview encompasses everything in the living universe, including animals, rocks, trees, caves, spirits, elemental forces, weather— whatever dwells in the hidden realms of lower, middle, or upper worlds. Shamanic practitioners believe that an individual's mental distress and/or physical ailment is rooted in imbalance with the natural order. This can be the result of soul loss, intrusions from other spiritual entities, curses, or trauma from physical, psychic, emotional, mental, spiritual, or even communal assault. Exploring the spiritual and transpersonal dialog with a shamanic practitioner has a history of use in both developed and less-developed parts of the world.

Treatments: What to Expect

A shamanic practitioner invites you into a ceremonial setting, in which sacred objects are ritually arranged, often with natural elements of fire or water or earth. They may induce a relaxation state through drumming or rattling or chanting, then move into non-ordinary states of consciousness to communicate with totem animals, spirit guides, or other cosmic or supernatural entities. These non-ordinary states allow the shaman to intercede for the individual seeking purification or healing. The co-journeyer may ask questions or be silent or be asked to receive certain blessings—depending on the historical lineage of the shaman. Some shamans from Peru and Ecuador will douse their seeker with flower essence by spraying it from their mouths, sometimes over a candle, or sometimes just on one's body or onto a central altar.

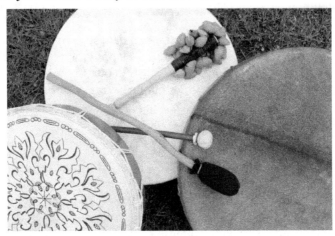

The three main activities of shamanic healing include journeying to non-ordinary realms to seek information or healing allies, extractions (working to remove spirits possession), and soul retrieval. Rituals for accessing these states of consciousness vary among societies, and include drumming, chanting, use of entheogenic (hallucinatory) plant mixtures such as ayahuasca, vision quests, and rapid breathwork. After the session or journey, the seeker may want to slowly integrate back into the everyday world by reflecting on the insights gained, journaling, or resting. Integration is an important component of any shamanic work, and guidance should be sought and followed.

Setting: In homes, clinics, private homes, or in nature.
Duration: One hour, to a day or several days.
Cost: Free, exchange, or $40–200 per session.

Best Suited for These Conditions

- Loss of meaning and purpose
- Unresolved grief
- Chronic mental distress
- Spiritual growth
- Divining future
- Contact with guardian spirits or totemic animal

- Physical healing with psycho-spiritual-emotional emphasis
- Communal healing
- Detoxification and purification
- Deconstructing an old identity and re-authoring a new story

Coaching Tip

It's been said that a shamanic journey is not for the faint of heart. Even when planning to go on a shamanic journey, much trepidation can precede it. Shamanic journeys are best led by shamans or shamanic practitioners who have learned their healing art through a rigorous process of training and initiation, or from a recognized educational program that includes certification from organizations such as the Foundation for Shamanic Studies. *Shamans in A Code of Ethics* has been created for shamanic healing practitioners and can serve as a guide for anyone s seeking this form of spiritual healing.

Contraindications

From a Western medical viewpoint, most licensed mental health counselors and psychotherapists would not recommend that individuals being treated for psychosis or dissociative states work with shamanic practitioners. They may also recommend that pregnant women or people with anxiety disorders avoid the intense exploratory work in shamanic rituals. However, this warning is not shared by those with alternative worldviews, such as, native healers throughout indigenous cultures, and even the psychiatrists and mental health counselors who work in medically pluralistic societies that honor indigenous healing modalities like the spiritism clinics and healing centers in Brazil and Peru. The growing numbers of Western-trained medical and health care practitioners who have sought shamanic training would also see the benefit of having a shaman attend to the social, psycho-emotional, and spiritual dimensions of mentally troubled individuals, a cultural approach that values collective healing as much if not more than individual therapy.

Research and Benefits

One of the most complete explorations of the therapeutic benefit of shamanic approaches is captured in the 25-year work of medical anthropologist and mental health counselor, Marlene Dobkin de Rios, PhD, in several books and papers, including *Brief Psychotherapy with the Latino Immigrant Client*. An expert on ayuahuasca use among native people in South America, she discussed how the shaman-assisted excursions into expanded states of consciousness brought about relief from anxiety, fears, agitation, pain, and stress-related illness among the seekers. The therapeutic alliance between shaman and participant can yield profound results in both self-awareness and psycho-emotional, spiritual, social, and physical healing. Other research by Lori Thayer examined how shamanic healing can be adopted into the biomedical health care system in the US (Thayer).

According to the Foundation of Shamanic Studies, *several* ongoing projects are dedicated to preserving the rich legacy of indigenous shamanism wherever indigenous traditions, people and habitats are threatened. A Code of Ethics was developed at the Foundation and can be found at shamanism.org/resources/FSSCodeEthics.pdf

Training and Credentials

Over the last 20 years, more health care practitioners who were conventionally trained in biomedicine (allopathy) are seeking shamanic training, sometimes for their own personal growth and development, but also for inclusion into their clinical practices. This syncretic (fusion of spiritual practice, folk healing and biomedicine) activity has been accused of cultural appropriation and commodification; however, systems of medical pluralism have existed for centuries, and there are conferences and organizations of "registered" traditional healers and shamans now working side-by-side, even in hospital environments, with conventional doctors. Because shamans can act as healers, counselors, arbitrators, and educators, most indigenous traditions require arduous training and initiation rites.

Shamans in Ecuador are closely tied to their communities, hear confessions, know who is been unjustly treated, seek restitution, facilitate forgiveness circles, and have socio-political influence. In indigenous shamanism, shamans are chosen by birthright and called by the spirit world.

Resources

Down to Earth: The Shaman's Circle—shamanscircle.com.
Dream Change (John Perkins)—dreamchange.org.
Embodied Shamanism: Shapeshifting into a New Narrative for Living a Life You Love, Residential retreat (Michael Stone)—welloflight.com
Foundation for Shamanic Studies (Michael and Sandra Harner)—shamanism.org.
The Four Winds Light Body Training (Alberto Villoldo)—thefourwinds.com.
Lynn Andrews Mystery School—lynnandrews.com/shaman-training.
Last Mask Center—lastmaskcenter.org.
Living Shaman Museum, founded by Connie Grauds, RPh, dedicated to educating about the living gifts of the Amazonian people for conservation and protection.

Pachamama Alliance, ongoing advocacy for personal and planetary
transformation, original efforts concentrated on indigenous rights of the
Achuar nation in Ecuador—pachamama.org
Power Soul Retrieval Training (Sandra Ingerman)—sandraingerman.com.
Three-Year Program of Advanced Initiations in Shamanism and Shamanic
Healing (Foundation of Shamanic Studies)—shamanism.org.

Bibliography
Black Elk, N. 2000. *Black Elk Speaks: Being the Life Story of a Holy Man
of the Oglala Sioux.* As told through John G. Neihardt (Flaming
Rainbow). 21st century ed. University of Nebraska Press.
Dobkin de Rios, M. *Brief Psychotherapy with the Latino Immigrant Client.*
Haworth Press; 2001.
Dioszegi, V. *Tracing Shamans in Siberia. The Story of an Ethnographical
Research Expedition.*Translated from the Hungarian by Aita Rajkay
Babo. Oosterhout, Anthropological Publications, 1968.
Ekrem, I & Mortensen, LB, eds. Peter Fisher, translator. *Historia
Norwegie.* Museum Tusculanum Press, 2003.
Eliade, M. *Shamanism: Archaic Techniques of Ecstacy.* Translated from
the French by Willard R. Trask. (Revised and enlarged from the
original French edition, *Le Charmanisme et les techniques archaiques
de l'extase,* 1951). Bollingen Foundation, 1964.
Halifax, J. *Shaman, the Wounded Healer.*Crossroad, 1982.
Harner, MJ. *The Way of the Shaman.* 3rd ed. Harper & Row, 1990.
Heinze, R-I. *Shamans of the 20th Century.* Irvington Publishers, 1991.
Keeney, B. *Shaking Medicine.* Inner Traditions, 2007.
Lyon, WS. *Encyclopedia of Native American Shamanism: Sacred
Ceremonies of North America.* ABC-CLIO. 1998.
Narby, J & Huxley, F, eds. . *Shamans through Time: 500 Years on the
Path to Knowledge.* JP Tarcher/Putnam, 2001.
Plotkin, MJ. *Tales of a Shaman's Apprentice: An Ethnobotanist Searches
for New Medicines in the Amazon Rain Forest.* Viking, 1993.
Thayer, LL. "The Adoption of Shamanic Healing into the Biomedical
Health Care System in the United States" (2009). Open Access
Dissertations. scholarworks.umass.edu/open_access_dissertations/60.
Accessed April, 2017.

TENSION AND TRAUMA RELEASE EXERCISES (TRE)
Elaine Santos

Tension and trauma release exercises (TRE®) are a series of movements that create a mild body tremor to release tension from the muscles.

History

TRE was created by David Berceli, PhD, in the late 1990s while working and living with large traumatized populations in Africa and the Middle East. Berceli was a relief worker with expertise in therapeutic bodywork and he observed a universal automatic physical response to stress; the contracting of the neck, shoulders, and ilio-psoas, which one might recognize as the fetal position. He also observed physical shaking occurring before, during, and after stressful situations. Berceli started his journey studying this shaking mechanism and uncovered a way to release the tension held in the muscles that contract during a stressful event. Because this response is part of the autonomic nervous system that controls the body's involuntary processes, he created exercises that fatigue those muscles and this results in mild tremoring that releases the held tension (Scaer IX-X). TRE is taught and trained worldwide.

Philosophy

We are genetically encoded to tremor. The exercises do not do anything to the body except reawaken and reengage this natural tremoring mechanism that has been dormant inside us.

—David Berceli

Humans naturally tremor when the autonomic nervous system is over-stimulated, whether in response to good or bad events. Examples include shaking from news of winning a large sum of money to experiencing a terrifying car accident. The use of tremoring or shaking as a healing technique is also not new. From the collective healing dances of the San people in Africa to Dine (Navajo) shamans in southwestern US, to people in Christian faiths who experience "speaking in tongues," and trembling practices in qigong and Kundalini yoga, involuntary movement as a spiritual and healing process has been part of many cultures for a long time (Schweitzer, 17-19).

The philosophy of TRE is based on the fundamental idea that stress, tension, and trauma is both psychological and physical (traumaprevention.com). Dr. Berceli took his observations of shaking and studied the meaning of tremors in the research of neurology, psychology, and physiology. Shaking or tremoring is often associated with neurological disorders or a way to diagnose psychological conditions, however in the world of physiology, since the 1900s, there has been research showing the positive effects of tremoring and how this can be applied to improve physical conditions and improve athletic performance. Instead of looking at tremors as part of a pathology of human neurophysiology Berceli believes a self-induced body tremor can be a way for the brain to down-regulate an over-excited system (Berceli 2015, 7).

Trauma and tension release exercises activate a shaking mechanism, which causes the muscles to relax. "TRE is taught purely as a neurophysiological process of deep relaxation that allows people to connect to themselves in a healthier manner." (Berceli 2015, 278) This deep relaxation can reduce stress in the spine, neck, shoulders, and pelvis. The exercises activate the relaxation response of the parasympathetic nervous system that decreases blood pressure, heart rate, and allows the body to digest and sleep. When tension is released anywhere in the body, the brain registers a reduction in pain signals, producing new hormones that promote healing (traumaprevention.com).

What is unique about this relaxation technique is it does not require conscious control of the body. TRE is working with the unconscious part of the brain so an individual can listen to music or even watch TV while their body releases tension.

Treatments: What to Expect
TRE is a self-help technique that can be learned by books, videos, by a practitioner individually or in a group setting, in-person or by videoconference.

It is recommended to take off shoes and socks to perform the exercises. The first five exercises target leg muscles; the next two exercises induce tremoring, first while standing and then in a supine position. After a period of time, to end the tremoring, leg muscles are contracted and released.

People who are new to TRE should tremor at a maximum fifteen minutes two to three times a week. It is important to not fatigue the muscles and to have self-regulation, which is defined by Berceli as the ability to recognize emotional overwhelm and be able to stop the shaking process.
Setting: Home or studio.
Duration: 35–55 minutes.
Cost: Group classes: $25–40, private sessions: $85–100.

Best Suited for These Conditions
- Muscle tension
- Chronic Stress and anxiety
- Insomnia
- PTSD

Coaching Tip

If your coaching clients want to learn TRE, you might consider asking them to look for a certified TRE practitioner through the TRE resources listed below. Even though TRE is a self-help technique and very easy to learn, it is recommended, especially for individuals with chronic conditions, to first work with a practitioner. TRE practitioners often have expertise in other professional fields such as psychology or yoga and can support the client and tailor the session to their needs. They should ask for personal references or talk to others who used this practitioner's services. TRE is a self-help technique that is used in conjunction with other therapies and should not replace medication or other treatments the client is currently using without the advice from their medical doctor or therapist.

Contraindications

Clients should consult their medical practitioner if they have a complex history of trauma or restricting physical or medical limitations before performing these exercises.

Individuals with the following conditions or who take medication for the following conditions should consult with a certified TRE provider to properly learn the technique and self-regulation:

- PTSD
- Depression and any mental illness or mental health issues
- Irregular blood pressure
- Hypo or hyperglycemia
- Epilepsy
- Sever chronic pain
- Recent surgery
- Pregnancy
- Broken bones, strains, or sprains

Research and Benefits

Although there is much anecdotal evidence regarding TRE, and many pilot clinical outcome studies are in process and have verified its efficacy around the globe, larger controlled quantitative and qualitative studies are needed (traumaprevention.com/research). Research studies and in-progress clinical studies featured on traumaprevention.com range from occupational health, military use, domestic violence, to stress and PTSD.

Practitioner Training and Credentials

There are four types of certification training programs:

- TRE® Certified Providers have completed the Global Certification Program, which has two modules and are certified to teach groups and individuals. TRE Certified Providers focus on teaching the exercises and supporting their students/clients through the processing of the experience.

- TRE® Certification Trainers have been personally invited by TRE, LLC, to become trainers and their responsibility is to educate, train, and certify TRE Certified Providers. Trainers provide face-to-face workshops, supervision, and oversight of requirements.
- TRE Agency Based Instructors are already working for an agency or organization. The certification is limited to teaching TRE within the agency, healthcare professionals have to be present during sessions, and several people from the agency are to be trained.
- TRE Provisionally Certified is a free certification for selected people who have been impacted by a large-scale disaster. The TRE Provisionally Certified can only teach in group settings with other co-trainers, and must teach for free to those affected by the disaster.

Many Certified TRE providers work in other professional fields and have a variety of specializations. It is the responsibility of the providers to work within their scope and it is the client's or student's responsibility to find a provider that fits their needs.

Resources
TRE®—traumaprevention.com
TRE Provider list—traumaprevention.com/tre-provider-list
Lumos Transforms—lumostransforms.com

References
Berceli, D. "A Letter from Dr. Berceli." traumaprevention.com/what-is-tre/get-tre-certifiedfrom-david-berceli. Accessed April 11, 2017.

Berceli, D. *Shake It Off Naturally.* CreateSpace Independent Publishing, 2015.

Brown, E. elizabethbrown.co.uk/what-i-do/tre. Accessed March 7, 2017.

Scaer, R. "Foreword." in David Berceli, *Shake It Off Naturally.* CreateSpace Independent Publishing, 2015.

Schweitzer, E. "Trembling with Joy: Anthropology and Trembling Practices Worldwide TRE." in David Berceli, *Shake It Off Naturally.* CreateSpace Independent Publishing, 2015.

Whole Systems

TRADITIONAL CHINESE MEDICINE
Kevonya Elzia

Traditional Chinese medicine is a whole system of medical practices originating in China and dating back over 2,000 years.

History
The origin of traditional Chinese medicine (TCM) can be traced back to 476-221 BCE (who.org). The roots of Chinese medicine philosophy began in Taoist mysticism and shamanistic practices, with later influences by Buddhist teachings (Gascoigne). Just prior to 1949 in China, TCM was at risk of being replaced by Western medicine as the dominant medical practice of choice. However, after the Communist government came into power in 1949, it was decided that TCM offered "a practical, simple and affordable system of healthcare that could be applied to all sections of the population" (Gascoigne). This revitalization of traditional medicine spilled over to China's neighbors and other eastern countries.

Philosophy
TCM is an integrative holistic system of medicine that acknowledges the mental, emotional, physical, social, environmental, and spiritual components of a person's life when attempting to address both the promotion and maintenance of wellbeing and the management of chronic conditions.

There are four key concepts in TCM. One is the concept of yin and yang, which in Chinese medicine is at the core of everything from the human body to the external environment. The concept of yin and yang represents the balance between the dual nature of our universe. Another key concept is qi (pronounced chee). Qi energy flows throughout the body in channels called meridians. Qi, together with blood, provides nourishment to the body and internal organs. The third key concept of TCM is the five internal organs that are the basis for all TCM diagnoses. The organs are heart, lung, spleen, liver, and kidney. Each of these organs acts as a central hub to corresponding areas of the body based on Chinese ideology. The fourth key concept is the five elements: fire, metal, wood, water, and earth. Fire connects to summer, metal connects to autumn, wood connects to spring, water connects to winter, and earth is at the center. Because of the belief that our internal and external environments are interconnected and interdependent, the five elements as well as the four seasons are taken into consideration when it comes to maintaining wellbeing.

The balance between yin and yang can be disrupted due to internal or external influences. The disruption results in qi and blood being unable to flow harmoniously, and produces symptoms of disharmony or, if left untreated, of illness. There are twelve main channels within the body, each associated with a particular organ. Along each channel there are acupuncture/acupressure points through which a practitioner can access the flow of qi and help both address the imbalance and treat the resulting illness. From this, the Chinese have been able to create a system of medicine that can effectively treat a wide range of disorders.

Treatments: What to Expect

Treatment can include one of the following interventions or a combination of them.

- Acupuncture
- Acupressure
- Cupping
- Herbal preparations
- Special diet instructions
- Qigong or tai chi exercises
- Meditation instruction
- Massage

Setting: Private room or group clinic.
Duration: 15–90 minutes.
Cost: $35–150 plus the cost of herbal preparations.

Best Suited for These Conditions

- Musculoskeletal disease
- Respiratory disease
- Circulatory disease
- Diseases of the digestive tract and related conditions
- Urogenital disease
- Gynecological disease
- Neurological disorders

Coaching Tip

Consider building your own network of TCM practitioners by calling local TCM colleges, asking trusted health care providers about their recommendations, and visiting their clinics to find out about their communication style, therapies, "bedside" manner, fees, services, and philosophy. Adding TCM into your own health care regimen can be a powerful preventive health measure. When you experience TCM yourself, you'll be more confident in talking about this remarkable healing system with interested clients.

Contraindications
Certain treatments and herbal preparations are not appropriate for administration during pregnancy.

Research and Benefits
The following research has shown that this modality has been beneficial for the following conditions:

Heart Health
Xu, Zhaoxia, et al. "Statistical Validation of Traditional Chinese Medicine Syndrome Postulates in the Context of Patients with Cardiovascular Disease." *Journal of Alternative and Complementary Medicine* 19, no. 10 (October 2013): 799-804. doi: 10.1089/acm.2012.0487.

Respiratory Health
Lin, Li Li, et al. "Application of Traditional Chinese Medical Herbs in Prevention and Treatment of Respiratory Syncytial Virus." *Evidence-Based Complementary and Alternative Medicine* (September 4, 2016): 1-13. doi: 10.1155/2016/6082729.

Lau, T. F., et al. "Using Herbal Medicine as a Means of Prevention Experience during the SARS Crisis." *American Journal of Chinese Medicine* 33, no. 3 (June 2005): 345-356.

Urinary Health
Christie, Connie L. "A Case Study on the Management of Benign Prostatic Hypertrophy Using Acupuncture and Chinese Herbal Medicine." *American Acupuncturist* 64 (Summer, 2013): 22-28.

Pain Management
Chen, Bo, et al. "Traditional Chinese Medications for Knee Osteoarthritis Pain: A Meta-Analysis of Randomized Controlled Trials." *American Journal of Chinese Medicine* 44, no. 4 (July, 2016): 677-703. doi: 10.1142/S0192415X16500373.

Digestive Health
"Chinese Herbal Treatment of Chronic Digestive Disorders." *Oriental Medicine Journal* 10, no. 4 (Fall 2002): 11-19.

Neurological Health
Dongman, Chao, et al. "From Acupuncture to Interaction between Δ-Opioid Receptors and Na+ Channels: A Potential Pathway to Inhibit Epileptic Hyperexcitability." *Evidence-Based Complementary and*

Alternative Medicine 2013 (January, 2013): 1-17. doi:
10.1155/2013/216016.
Naizhao Li, Lance. "Treating Migraine Headache with Acupuncture."
American Acupuncturist 67, (Spring 2014): 34.

Reproductive Health
Azizi, Hoda, et al. "Menopause-Related Symptoms: Traditional Chinese
Medicine versus Hormone Therapy." *Alternative Therapies in Health
and Medicine* 17, no. 4 (July/August 2011): 48-53.
Baccetti, Sonia, et al. "Acupuncture and Traditional Chinese Medicine for
Hot Flushes in Menopause: A Randomized Trial." *Journal of
Alternative and Complementary Medicine* 20, no. 7 (July, 2014): 550-
557. doi: 10.1089/acm.2012.0499.
Cahill, Kandace. "A Benign Complex Ovarian Cyst Treated with
Traditional Chinese Medicine: A Case Study." *American Acupuncturist*
58 (Winter 2012): 24-36.
Sai, Kong, et al. "The Complementary and Alternative Medicine for
Endometriosis: A Review of Utilization and Mechanism." *Evidence-
Based Complementary and Alternative Medicine* (January 2014): 1-16.
doi: 10.1155/2014/146383.

Practitioner Training and Credentials

TCM practitioners are required to complete a total of 2,460 hours of
training that consists of at least 1,560 hours of theory and
laboratory/clinical practice and 900 hours of supervised clinical practicum.
These programs are typically based in a college or university setting and
take three to four years to complete when attending full-time.

Health professionals who are trained in other modalities of healing,
such as Western medicine, can become licensed in TCM, but are required
to complete formal training at an institution that specializes in TCM
training and must complete the necessary laboratory and supervised
clinical practicum hours.

Resources

World Health Organization—who.org
Institute of Traditional Medicine—itmonline.org
Institute of Qigong & Integrative Medicine—iqim.org
Shen Nong—shen-nong.com

References

World Health Organization. *Benchmarks for Training in Traditional Complementary and Alternative Medicine.* World Health Organization, 2010.

Gascoigne, S. *The Chinese Way to Health: A Self-Help Guide to Traditional Chinese Medicine.* Charles E. Tuttle Company, 1997.

"Holistic Concept of Chinese Medicine." shen-nong.com. Accessed March 30, 2017.

"TCM History–Introduction." shen-nong.com. Accessed March 30, 2017.

TRADITIONAL EAST ASIAN MEDICINE
Kevonya Elzia

Traditional East Asian Medicine refers to the traditional systems of healing originating in China, Japan, Korea, and throughout South Asian countries.

History
Many Asian medical modalities are connected to traditional Chinese medicine (TCM) in some way due to the strong influence TCM had in the East Asian region of the world. Despite the original influence of TCM, each country adapted the Chinese medical model to the values and needs of the country's people. Two of the medical systems included in this category of East Asian medicine are traditional Japanese medicine, also known as Kampo, which took root in Japan in 808 CE (kampo.ca); and traditional Korean medicine (TKM), which includes Sasang Medicine, a system of care in Korea that was established in the 1800s (Wagman, G., 2016). Other East Asian medical systems include: Vietnamese traditional medicine, Tibetan medicine, traditional Mongolian medicine, and traditional medicine of Bhutan.

Philosophy
As each of these medical systems has been adapted to the needs of the region in which it is practiced, the philosophy of each varies. Unique to Korean Oriental medicine (KOM) is its "...theory that a microsystem [of the body] is found on the hands. In a microsystem, the whole body is reflected in just one area such as the ear, hand, or scalp. Conditions of the body, wherever they might be, from head to toe, can be treated by using points in one microsystem." (Richards).

Sasang medicine, which is a part of TKM theory of practice, is based on a philosophy that believes that "human matters influence the physiological and pathological conditions" (Junghee). It also highlights the importance of taking individual variability into account when treating patients.

A review of Kampo reveals that it uses many of the theories and principles of TCM, but also has incorporated abdominal palpation as an additional method of diagnosing conditions. Also, Kampo uses a different group of primary herbs than those utilized in TCM.

Treatments: What to Expect

Like TCM, treatment can include one or a combination of the following interventions:

- Acupuncture
- Acupressure
- Herbal preparations
- Special dietary instructions
- Cupping
- Meditation instruction
- Massage

Setting: Private room or in a group clinic.
Duration: 15 to 90 minutes.
Cost: $35–150 plus the cost of herbal preparations.

Best Suited for These Conditions

- Migraines
- Muscle tension
- Depression
- Arthritis
- Pain management
- Digestive health
- Respiratory health
- Dental health
- Reproductive health
- Urinary health

Coaching Tip

Facilitate your client's exploration to find respected and highly recommended practitioners. Use the resources below and build your own network of reliable and caring professionals in traditional East Asian medicine.

Contraindications

Certain treatments and herbal preparations are not appropriate for administration during pregnancy

Research and Benefits

The following research has shown that this modality has been beneficial for the following conditions:

Pain

Arai, Young-Chang P., et al. "Effects of Kamishoyosan, a Traditional Japanese Kampo Medicine, on Pain Conditions in Patients with Intractable Persistent Dentoalveolar Pain Disorder." *Evidence-Based Complementary & Alternative Medicine* (October 1, 2015): 1-5. doi: 10.1155/2015/750345.

Arai, Young-Chang, et al. "Integration of a Kampo Medicine, Nijutsuto, and Western Medical Treatment in the Treatment of Long-Term Frozen Shoulder Refractory to Western Medical Treatment: A Case Series." *Journal of Evidence-Based Complementary & Alternative Medicine* 20, no. 2 (April 2015): 157-161. doi: 10.1177/2156587214568346.

Hijikata, Yasuyo, et al. "Two Kampo Medicines, Jidabokuippo and Hachimijiogan, Alleviate Sprains, Bruises and Arthritis." *Evidence-Based Complementary and Alternative Medicine* 4, no. 4 (December 2007): 463-467. doi: 10.1093/ecam/ne1105.

Nishimura, Ko, et al. "Complete Recovery from Tension-Type Headache through Kampo Medicine." *Journal of Alternative and Complementary Medicine* 15, no. 7 (July 2009): 799-801. doi: 10.1089/acm.2008.0538.

Cancer Complications (with Western medicine)

Jun-ichi, Yamakawa, et al. "Significance of Kampo, Traditional Japanese Medicine, in Supportive Care of Cancer Patients." *Evidence-Based Complementary and Alternative Medicine* (January 2013): 1-10. doi: 10.1155/2013/746486.

Digestive

Kori, Kazuyoshi, et al. "Go-Rei-San, a Kampo Medicine, Reduces Postoperative Nausea and Vomiting: A Prospective, Single-Blind, Randomized Trial." *Journal of Alternative and Complementary Medicine* 19, no. 12 (December 2013): 946-950. doi: 10.1089/acm.2013.0118.

Oikawa, Tetsuro, et al. "Hangekobokuto (Banxia-Houpo-Tang), a Kampo Medicine That Treats Functional Dyspepsia." *Evidence-Based Complementary and Alternative Medicine* 6, no. 3 (September 2009): 375-378. doi: 10.1093/ecam/nem101.

Sachiko, Mogami and Hattori Tomohisa. "Beneficial Effects of Rikkunshito, a Japanese Kampo Medicine, on Gastrointestinal Dysfunction and Anorexia in Combination with Western Drug: A Systematic Review." *Evidence-Based Complementary and Alternative Medicine* (January 2014): 1-7. Accessed through EBSCO*host*, doi: 10.1155/2014/519035.

Woong, Kim, et al. "Anti-Viral Effect of Herbal Medicine Korean Traditional Cynanchum Paniculatum (Bge.) Kitag Extracts." *African*

Journal of Traditional, Complementary and Alternative Medicines 14, no. 3 (July 2017): 194-198. doi: 10.21010/ajtcam.v14i3.21.

Cold/Flu

Takayuki, Nagai, et al. "Alleviative Effects of a Kampo (A Japanese Herbal) Medicine 'Maoto (Ma-Huang-Tang)' on the Early Phase of Influenza Virus Infection and its Possible Mode of Action." *Evidence-Based Complementary and Alternative Medicine* (January 2014): 1-12. doi: 10.1155/2014/187036.

Dental Health

Hideki, Okamoto, et al. "A Valid Approach in Refractory Glossodynia: A Single-Institution 5-Year Experience Treating with Japanese Traditional Herbal (Kampo) Medicine." *Evidence-Based Complementary and Alternative Medicine* (January 2013): 1-8. doi: 10.1155/2013/354872.

Liao, James, et al. "Effects of Japanese Traditional Herbal Medicines (Kampo) on Growth and Virulence Properties of Porphyromonas Gingivalis and Viability of Oral Epithelial Cells." *Pharmaceutical Biology* 51, no. 12 (December 2013): 1538-1544. doi: 10.3109/13880209.2013.801995.

Eye Health

Hayasaka, Seiji, et al. "Traditional Japanese Herbal (Kampo) Medicines and Treatment of Ocular Diseases: A Review." *American Journal of Chinese Medicine* 40, no. 5 (October 2012): 887-904. doi: 10.1142/S0192415X12500668.

Ju-Hyun, Jeon, et al. "Acupuncture Reduces Symptoms of Dry Eye Syndrome: A Preliminary Observational Study." *Journal of Alternative and Complementary Medicine* 16, no. 12 (December 2010): 1291-1294. doi: 10.1089/acm.2009.0537.

Respiratory Health

Kim, Ki-Suk, et al. "Effects of the Inhaled Treatment of Liriope Radix on an Asthmatic Mouse Model." *American Journal of Chinese Medicine* 43, no. 3 (May 2015): 425-441. doi: 10.1142/S0192415X15500275.

Kyun Ha, Kim, et al. "Therapeutic Effect of Chung-Pae, an Experimental Herbal Formula, on Acute Lung Inflammation Is Associated with Suppression of NF-Kb and Activation of Nrf2." *Evidence-Based Complementary and Alternative Medicine* (January 2013): 1-11. doi: 10.1155/2013/659459.

Nagai, Takayuki, et al. "Proteomic Analysis of Anti-Inflammatory Effects of a Kampo (Japanese Herbal) Medicine 'Shoseiryuto (Xiao-Qing-Long-Tang)' on Airway Inflammation in a Mouse Model." *Evidence-

Based Complementary and Alternative Medicine 8, no. 1 (January 2011): 1-13. doi: 10.1093/ecam/nep151.

Postpartum Health
Ushiroyama, Takahisa, et al. "Efficacy of the Kampo Medicine Xiong-Gui-Tiao-Xue-Yin (Kyuki-Chouketsu-In), a Traditional Herbal Medicine, in the Treatment of Maternity Blues Syndrome in the Postpartum Period." American Journal of Chinese Medicine 33, no. 1 (January 2005): 117-126.

Practitioner Training and Credentials

Currently, there is not a formal college- or university-based curriculum that focuses solely on Kampo or KOM. Even in Japan it is a specialization that is added to the primary curriculum. Practitioners should have at least taken a course that has focused on the principles of Kampo or KOM, and preferably have studied under a mentor skilled in Kampo or KOM to obtain clinical experience.

Resources

Institute of Traditional Medicine—itmonline.org
Kampo Japanese Traditional Medicine and Therapeutics—kampo.ca
Oriental Medicine Journal—omjournal.com
Evidence Based Complementary and Alternative Medicine Journal—hindawi.com/journals/ecam

References

Gascoigne, S. *The Chinese Way to Health: A Self-Help Guide to Traditional Chinese Medicine.* Charles E. Tuttle Company, 1997.
Institute of Traditional Medicine. itmonline.org. Accessed March 31. 2017.
Jong Yeol, K, et al. "Comparison of Sasang Constitutional Medicine, Traditional Chinese Medicine and Ayurveda." *Evidence-Based Complementary and Alternative Medicine* 8, no. 1 (January 2011): 1-6. , doi: 10.1093/ecam/neq052.
Junghee, Y, et al. "Sasang Constitutional Medicine and Traditional Chinese Medicine: A Comparative Overview." *Evidence-Based Complementary and Alternative Medicine* 2012 (January 2012): 1-17. , doi: 10.1155/2012/980807.
Kampo Japanese Traditional Medicine and Therapeutics. kampo.ca.
Korean Culture and Information Service (KOCIS). "An Ancient Medical Tradition." Korea.net. Accessed March 31. 2017.
Richards, A. "Why You've Never Heard of Korean Medicine." *Epoch Times*. December 1, 2015. Access.
Wagman, G. "The Korean Tradition of Sasang Medicine: Historical and Philosophical Perspectives." *Oriental Medicine Journal* 24, no. 5 (Late summer, 2016): 6-14.

WELLNESS INVENTORY
Jim Strohecker

The Wellness Inventory is an online, whole person assessment and life-balance program designed to promote sustainable improvement in people's lives and to maximize their capacity for personal wellbeing and optimal living.

History
The Wellness Inventory was first published as a booklet in 1975 by John Travis, concurrent with his opening the first wellness center in the United States (Mill Valley, CA). It supported the Wellness Resource Center's innovative program for personal lifestyle change, which focused on self-responsibility and engaged the whole person—body, mind, emotions, and spirit.

The field of coaching had not yet been defined in the 70s, but staff facilitators worked with clients' assessment results, much as coaches today work with clients, using a client-centered, empowered approach.

After many thousands of the booklet version had been used around the world, in 2001, the Inventory became an integrated, online program offering many features that couldn't be done by paper.

Philosophy
The Wellness Inventory program is rooted in three key wellness concepts developed by Dr. Travis in the 1970s.

Key Concept #1: The Illness-Wellness Continuum

> *Wellness is a process, never a static state.*
> —Wellness Workbook

Most of us assume that the absence of illness indicates wellness. There are actually many degrees of wellness, just as there are many degrees of illness. Besides this wide range of states of health, the Continuum illustrates the relationship between the treatment paradigm and the wellness paradigm, as shown by the inset arrows in the illustration in Foreword. An individual can move along the Continuum from a lack of illness, to beyond its Neutral Point into increasingly higher levels of wellness.

Key Concept #2: Iceberg Model of Heath and Disease

Illness and health are only the tip of the iceberg. To understand their causes you need to look beneath the surface.

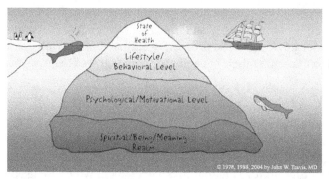

Your current state of health, be it one of disease or vitality, is just like the tip of the iceberg. This is the apparent, visible portion. If you don't like your state of health, you can attempt to change it, chiseling away at an unwanted condition such as weight. But, like an iceberg, as you chip away one part, more of the same rises to the surface. For true whole person life-balance and wellbeing, you need to address the deeper layers.

Key Concept #3: Wellness Energy System

Humans are all energy transformers, connected with the whole universe. All our life processes, including illness, depend upon how we manage energy.

We are open systems. We take in energy from all the sources around us, organize it, transform it, and return it to our environment. The efficient flow of energy is essential to wellness. Disease can be seen as the result of any interference to this flow.

The Wellness Energy System is represented by a wheel with twelve sections or dimensions (see Wellness Energy Wheel illustration in Foreword)—each of which represents a form of energy utilized in a basic life process. Three of these, Breathing, Eating, and Sensing, are inputs of energy. Eight others, Moving, Feeling, Thinking, Playing & Working, Communicating, Intimacy, Finding Meaning, and Transcending are the kinds of energy we return to the environment. The first section, Self-Responsibility & Love, is the context within which the wellness process best flourishes.

How we manage these primary life processes, in large part determines our own level of energy as well as our personal health of wellbeing.

Practice: What to Expect

The Wellness Inventory has the best results when used with clients who are open to exploring new possibilities for improvement, growth and an enhanced level of wellbeing in their lives.

Your client can take the Inventory on their own and work with you, or obtain coaching from a member of the network of Certified Wellness Inventory Coaches. Regardless, they need to allow at 45-60 minutes of quality time to complete the assessment, view their Wellbeing and Motivation Profiles, and then create their first action step.

The self-assessment portion is comprised of participants' responses to ten wellness statements in each of the twelve dimensions shown in the Wheel above. To each statement, they indicate how true this statement currently is in their life. They then indicate how motivated they are to increase their level of wellness represented by that statement in the next 30-60 days.

Both answers are rated on a Likert scale of 0–10. The assessment requires 30–40 minutes to complete with the ability to save their results and log off, returning later to complete it.

Wellness Statement	How True?	How Motivated to Improve?
I enjoy and take time for spontaneous activities.	2	9
I value myself for who I am, not just for what I do.	6	4
I avoid taking on unnecessary and unrealistic burdens and responsibilities.	4	8
I make an effort to play and work cooperatively, not competitively.	7	4

Upon completing the assessment, participants are presented with their Wellbeing Profile and their Motivation Profile for all twelve dimensions (see "Self-Assessed Wheel" illustration in Preface).

They are next asked to create their first action steps in a few of the areas where they had a low score and high level of motivation. They also have the option to have email reminders about their actions steps sent.

The participants are then directed to their Personal Wellness Home Page, their point of access for the rest of the year-long process their subscription provides, where they can use features that focus on raising their wellness awareness and improving their level of personal health and wellbeing.

A central feature of the program, the action plan includes an interactive virtual coach tool to help in creating action steps as well as to help refine the steps to be more realistic and doable (the SMART Step Process). Besides the email reminders for accountability, a progress tracker aids in their successful integration into their life.

Additional features include a reassessment at regular intervals, deeper learning on each dimension through the Study Center, a Resource Center of additional tools, and an online journal to record insights and experiences in each of the twelve dimensions.

Setting: Any quiet location with Internet access.
Duration: 45–60 minutes.
Cost: $39.95/one year subscription.

Best Suited for These Conditions

- Stress
- Chronic pain
- Hypertension
- Type II diabetes and pre-diabetes
- Heart disease
- Stroke
- Cancer
- Addiction recovery
- Burnout
- Compassion fatigue
- Obesity
- Promotion of heart and brain health
- Promotion of resiliency

Coaching Tip

Coaches can recommend the Wellness Inventory program to clients they believe will benefit from broadening their current perspective to a more dynamic, comprehensive, whole person view of their lifestyle, behavior, and mindset.

It is also useful to clients experiencing a chronic illness and want to build their wellness awareness and skills in developing more effective self-care and internal self-management.

Contraindications

- serious mental health issues
- severe depression,
- serious cognitive decline
- serious addictions.

Research and Benefits

Based on twelve years' of experiences of Certified Wellness Inventory Coaches and other coaches working with the instrument, there have been positive results with individuals with a wide range of chronic conditions, particularly those most impacted by stress and lifestyle factors. The instrument is only recently becoming more widely accepted, which will attract peer-reviewed studies.

Two pilot programs, funded by insurance companies and delivered by hospitals in Arizona and Nebraska to employee populations, showed significant reduction in health risks as well as significant improvements in all biometrics tracked through pre- and post-health risk appraisals and physicals, including blood pressure, total cholesterols, triglycerides, weight loss, BMI, and frequency of exercise. The programs consisted of a workshop series on the twelve dimensions of wellness, pre- and post-Wellness Inventory assessments, and use of the Wellness Inventory program's behavioral change features throughout.

A pilot program to train Sexual Assault Response Coordinators (SARCs) from the US Military Academy at West Point and other Army bases was based on the Wellness Inventory and a series of fourteen weekly face-to-face advocacy sessions that focused on the twelve dimensions with victims of sexual assault.

In use of the Wellness Inventory with college students in academic courses there is evidence that the program may be an effective tool for reducing student anxiety and stress, as well as improving sleep and concentration.

Practitioner Training and Credentials
There are two levels of certification for coaches: Wellness Inventory Certification Training consists of two levels: The Wellness Inventory Certification Training is delivered in two levels. Level I Certification Training is fourteen weeks. Level II Certification Training (Holographic Coaching Practicum) is a seven-week training to deepen coaching skills using the Holographic Growth Process as well as the Coaching Core Competencies. Both are delivered via live phone teleconferencing 2 hours per week.

Resources
Wellness Inventory Program—wellpeople.com.
Wellness Inventory Certification Training—certifywelness.com.

Bibliography
Arloski, M, *Wellness Coaching for Lasting Lifestyle Change*, Whole Person Associates, 2007.

Firth, KM. and Smith, K. "A Survey of Multi-Dimensional Health and Fitness Indexes," *Military Medicine* August 2010. 175, 111–113.

Palombi, BJ. "Psychometric Properties of Wellness Instruments", *Journal of Counseling & Development*, 71 (Nov-Dec 1992): 221-225.

SRI International, *Spas and the Global Wellness Market: Synergies and Opportunities*, SRI International, 2010, iii, 5, 19, 59.

Travis, JW & Ryan, RS. *Wellness Workbook. How to Achieve Enduing Health and Vitality*. Celestial Arts, 2004.

Travis, JW, & Callander, MG. Wellness for Helping Professionals: Creating Compassionate Cultures. Wellness Associates Publications. 1990.